TWITCH

TWITCH

MY LIFE WITH PARKINSON'S: A MEMOIR

ANNMARIE O'CONNOR

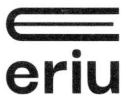

First published in the UK in 2025 by Eriu
An imprint of Bonnier Books UK
5th Floor, HYLO, 105 Bunhill Row,
London, EC1Y 8LZ

Copyright © Annmarie O'Connor, 2025

All rights reserved.

No part of this publication may be reproduced, stored or transmitted in any form or by any means, electronic, mechanical, photocopying or otherwise, without the prior written permission of the publisher.

The right of Annmarie O'Connor to be identified as Author of this work has been asserted by her in accordance with the Copyright, Designs and Patents Act, 1988.

A CIP catalogue record for this book is available from the British Library.

Trade Paperback ISBN: 978-1-80418-787-6

Also available as an ebook and an audiobook

1 3 5 7 9 10 8 6 4 2

Design and Typeset by IDSUK (Data Connection) Ltd
Printed and bound in Great Britain by Clays Ltd, Elcograf S.p.A.

Every reasonable effort has been made to trace copyright holders of material reproduced in this book, but if any have been inadvertently overlooked the publishers would be glad to hear from them.

This book is a work of Non-Fiction. Some names may have been changed to respect the privacy of those mentioned.

The authorised representative in the EEA is
Bonnier Books UK (Ireland) Limited.
Registered office address: Floor 3, Block 3, Miesian Plaza,
Dublin 2, D02 Y754, Ireland
compliance@bonnierbooks.ie
www.bonnierbooks.co.uk

To Andy
"Let me just stop you there..."

CONTENTS

INTRODUCTION		1
CHAPTER ONE	**Twitch** How it starts	3
CHAPTER TWO	**Diagnosis** The news	35
CHAPTER THREE	**Drugs** One size does not fit all	53
CHAPTER FOUR	**Headlines** I'm coming out	81
CHAPTER FIVE	**Grief** Goodbye, old life	97
CHAPTER SIX	**Rebel Yell** Anger is an energy	107
CHAPTER SEVEN	**Miracles** Persistence pays	129

CHAPTER EIGHT	**Side Effects** Here we go again	155
CHAPTER NINE	**Full Circle** Lessons learned	175
CHAPTER TEN	**Acceptance** Life goes on	193

Epilogue   209
Acknowledgements   211
About Annmarie   213

AUTHOR'S NOTE

The information I share in this book is based on my personal experience and treatment of Parkinson's. If you or someone you know suspects they might have symptoms of the disease, please contact your primary healthcare provider.

INTRODUCTION

I'M HERE TO TAKE you on a journey between two points in my life – before and after. In between is a fleeting moment that radically altered who I am and how I move through the world. Blink and you miss it: a twitch.

From the outside, a lot still looks the same. I work in the same industry, I live in the same place, I surround myself with the same people. But I am not the same, and I will never be the same again. An unexpected Parkinson's diagnosis saw fit to that. For those of you who aren't familiar with the disease, don't worry – I wasn't either. I thought Parkinson's, with its characteristic stoop, shake and shuffle, affected men in their senior years, not women in their forties like me. It's safe to say I knew nothing. That would soon change.

Without giving away too much of my story here, let's say that my experience of living with an interloper who sought to scupper my motivation, mood and means of making a living was challenging. Because of this, it was clear I had to make a choice. I could play it small and stoic and 'manage' my condition, or I could share my medical coming-out story and, in doing so, help others who might feel similarly broken. I'm no expert, but this much I know: when something falls apart, whether it's your health, relationship or career, all rubble looks the same. Our humanity connects us, not our circumstances.

With that, I hope my path will guide, comfort, or give you a much-needed laugh as you navigate your own, wherever it might take you.

As for the twitch? It might be how this all starts, but it's certainly not how it ends. The story is mine to tell. And so, it begins ...

CHAPTER ONE
Twitch
How it starts

September 2020

I'M LYING IN BED, casting off the last remnants of sleep. My right arm stretches across the adjacent pillow. It feels heavy – sore, almost. As I push my body into a sitting position, my shoulder begins to ache. *God, it hurts.* I take a moment to recall what may have caused it. I was working on a photoshoot earlier in the week, thanks to a loosening of COVID-19 restrictions. *Maybe I pulled a muscle carrying those suitcases and garment bags by myself?* Still, I don't remember having felt any pain, not even a twinge until now. This is my first career-related injury, bar an iffy case of carpal tunnel at London Fashion Week a few years back. *Not bad innings for a 47-year-old.* With that, I put on my dressing gown and slippers, take two ibuprofen and prepare to go about my morning. Two suitcases still stand beside the wardrobe in my sister's guest bedroom. They're not going anywhere. Nor am I, by the looks of it. *Maybe today will be different,* I tell myself, knowing better, of course.

I'm viewing an apartment in Ballsbridge that looks decent, although I'll reserve judgement. Why I bother is anyone's guess. Most of what's available these days are real estate catfish or online scams, using pandemic restrictions to swindle deposits from unsuspecting renters. I wait with three couples in the mahogany foyer of what was desirable property a few decades ago. A man in a pink shirt arrives, his left ear cradling an iPhone. He points his right forefinger and thumb like a gun at us, seven masked strangers, before gesturing to the phone as he nods and makes *uh-huh* noises. He turns his back to the group, still making indeterminate sounds. *Is he . . . ? Are we . . . ?*

"Sorry about that," he says, looking at no one in particular. "You're all here, I assume, for number . . ." He points the gun again, looking for answers.

"88."

"Right, yeah." Happy with the joint confession, he puts the gun into his pocket and removes a folded face covering. "Remember, people *live* in this building, you know. So, try and, like, be as quiet as you can."

Before turning on his heel to adjust the belt on his skinny jeans (a portal to another era when denim cling film was borderline acceptable), I spot them. *Are those? Surely not. Brown winklepickers and white socks? Rule of thumb: never trust a man in pointier shoes than my stilettos. Would it be too obvious if I left now? Save us all some time?*

So-called fashion expert or not, I remind myself I'm in no position to judge anyone and ought to get on with things. My shoulder smarts in agreement. *Ouch.* Point taken.

As the other six follow the Pied Piper of Poor Choices up the stairwell, I pull up at the rear, spotting peeling paint, broken windowpanes and random shards of glass. Delightful. All that's missing is the police tape. Pulling out the world's noisiest set of keys, the pink shirt (who clearly doesn't do introductions) mumbles as he tries each of the metal skeletons before finally opening the door.

"Guys, figure it out amongst yourselves, but you might want to view it one or two at a time," he advises while still holding his mask.

It is clear to me why Dublin rentals have such strict pet policies: you can't swing a cat in most of them. I try to remain open-minded as I inspect the would-be crime scene. The dead plants are a special touch.

"As you can see, it's really spacious," says the pink shirt.

"What about safety?" I ask, spotting him inspecting the lock on the door handle.

"Yeah, that too."

Ah, master of the hard sell!

The couple beside me whisper like they're on a game show, careful not to reveal their strategy. I feel sick. The weight of my naivety crushes what self-esteem remains after seven months of lockdown. *I gave up a home I love and the seeds of a life in Cork. And for what? To live in my sister's guest room. To have my earnings dry up overnight. The one photoshoot I was permitted to style left me with a frozen shoulder. And those corporate dressing seminars I launched are now useless. Most people are working from home in their pyjamas, for God's sake. This bloody Zoom nonsense means I needn't have moved at all.* I can feel the blood draining from my face. It's too much. I need to leave.

"So, any thoughts?" asks the pink shirt, not even bothering to disguise the broken door lock.

"Disappointed," I reply. "It's not what I expected." This may be true, in part, but what disappoints me most is not staying put in Cork, not trusting my gut that I could be self-sufficient, not fighting to make it work, not believing in myself. I'm the disappointment.

He glances down at his winklepickers. "That's fair."

* * *

Looking back on the past seven months, no one could have predicted what happened: a global pandemic that forced the world to pause and hold its breath. Cue a never-ending stay-at-home order, slashed budgets, work opportunities reduced to the size of a video screen and me wondering what the hell I did.

Dublin and I weren't strangers. I've lived here twice before. No stranger to moving either, I was born in New York, grew up in Galway and I've worked and studied in London, Bologna and Monza, but of all the places I found myself, Cork is the city that anchored me. It's my adopted home.

My short-sighted thinking was that I would get more work in Dublin (or so I told myself) and a suitable place to live – the housing crisis notwithstanding. My longtime friend Andy suggested I store my belongings at his place, while my eldest sister, Margaret, happy to have me for an interim stay, offered her guest room while I got sorted. Three weeks and a state of emergency later, she and I became bubble buddies.

To say the early days of the pandemic were a test of our sisterly bond is an understatement. Related by blood, sure, but we may as well speak different languages. As the director of a financial services company, Margaret spent lockdown dealing with corporate bigwigs in kitchen video conferences, while I mainlined CBD oil and panic-filled the pantry with end-of-days vigour. Why doom scroll when you can be a doomsday prepper? Tinned fruit, rice pudding and custard – surely, there's some mention of trifle in the Book of Revelations? Not one to trifle, Margaret had no bandwidth for existential dread (or my talk of astrology and the universe), yet she would always turn up the radio when she heard a banger from The Rolling Stones or AC/DC, forcing me to dance with her. *I hate dancing.* The more I resisted, the more she persisted, flailing her arms and bandying her legs, determined to make me laugh or disown her – whichever came first. We may not always understand each other, but that was her way of telling me not to worry. Big corporate job, sure, but she is also a big softie.

Seasons passed and life stood still; our nerves frayed and patience thinned. So I looked for apartments and wrote fashion features about 'dopamine dressing' from the chest of drawers in Margaret's guest bedroom while she dealt with three-letter acronyms in her virtual boardroom. We were in suspended animation. Suspended by regret that I could make such a rookie move. Suspended by guilt that she couldn't do anything to help me. There is no blame here, only a good story when we look back and realise we got through it without losing our will to live. That said, the quicker I could find my own place, the more likely that story would become a reality. If she made me dance one more time, I'd crack up.

October 2020

Not long after the viewing, I get a call about a work opportunity – styling another photoshoot in Cork. Of course. The turnaround is quick due to Level 5 lockdown restrictions on the horizon. Can I be at the River Lee Hotel by Friday? Quicker than you can say "Irony is the universe's way of telling you that Cork *really* is the Real Capital" and that you messed up by moving. *Girl, I know. I know.*

Later that week, I am preparing the final looks in the hotel before model fittings begin. Today's shoot is about embracing comfort – chunky boots, knitted dresses and cosy layers – as we settle into another winter at home.

A lump in my throat forms as I look out from the third floor at Sunday's Well – a fashionable suburb of Cork hanging on the banks of the River Lee. Someone told me it was once a place of pilgrimage long associated with healing – a place of miracles.

I am tempted to draw the blinds. *Knock, knock.* Layla, our makeup artist, pops in for a socially distanced briefing, her apron filled with fifty fluffy, feathery and angled brushes. I'm always impressed at how she remembers which one does what and why. Amid talk of smoky eyes, dewy skin and the latest on her engagement, she takes a moment to check in with me.

"Look, this might be none of my business, but I just wanted to see if everything's alright, like? You're not really yourself today."

"Well, apart from a wonky shoulder from the last shoot I styled, I'm grand," I laugh, holding onto the clothes rail for support. "More on that later."

"OK so," she nods, upbeat but unconvinced. "Usually you're in your element with all these divine clothes, but look, we're all entitled to an off day."

"Goes without saying," she adds, "but if you need an ear, you know where I am."

Some people have therapist energy. Layla is one of them. Before she makes it to the door, the oversharing starts. It's out of my control. In about six-and-a-half minutes and, without warning, I recap each episode of The Biggest Mistake of My Life, distilling the main plot points into one concise sentence: "And so, I want to move back."

"Ah, that's a no-brainer. Call your letting agent, girl. Tell her the wind blew you back. Sure, we'll be standing here with open arms!"

On my break, I call my real estate contact about available units in my former apartment block. She tells me there are none free at present but will keep me in mind, even though the likelihood is slim, considering the current public health crisis.

The next day, fate intervenes. One of her tenants leaves suddenly for personal reasons, forgoing his security deposit. I am free to view the apartment and move in as soon as it is deep-cleaned, in line with COVID-19 protocols. "I can't believe it," she says, referring to our conversation less than 24 hours previous. "These things rarely happen." I agree to move in two weeks later just as the government reinstates Level 5 restrictions. My luck, for a change, couldn't be better. Unprecedented times, indeed.

October 31, 2020

A neon reminder glows in the dark: it's 3 a.m. I can't sleep thanks to the dull pain in my shoulder, which radiates down my arm. Too tired to bother finding my phone or the overhead light, I trudge to the bathroom in zombie mode, arms outstretched, hoping my hands will hit any sharp edges before my face does. The last thing I need is a broken nose and a bum shoulder when moving back to Cork this morning.

Not wanting to wake Margaret with the clackity bathroom light fan, I locate the medicine cabinet and find what I believe is a sachet of dissolvable paracetamol tablets along with a plastic cup. Plonk, fizz, gulp, swallow, regret.

The bathroom light screams as I fumble for the box of painkillers. *Poison. This must be poison.* Not quite. Milton Sterilising Tablets, actually. "Kills 99.9 per cent of germs" says the pink strapline and, according to the fine print, is potentially harmful to aquatic mammals. I begin to choke, panic and make violent hissing noises like a cat dislodging a furball. Convinced of my imminent and undignified end, I bang on Margaret's bedroom door.

"What?" a voice snaps in the darkness.

"Mags, I think I poisoned myself—"

No answer.

"—with Milton. The box says it's harmful to aquatic mammals. Maybe we should call A&E."

Still no answer.

The light goes on. Within seconds, Margaret stands in front of me fully robed and arms crossed, which, to her credit, is a rather impressive time-management skill.

"Are you an aquatic mammal?"

"No," I squeak, holding my throat.

"You don't seem sure."

Such a ninja move. I've got to admire it. Margaret could make a killing in the corporate seminar game – *Master Effective Boardroom Communication with the Art of the Rhetorical Question*. She looks ready to kill me.

"Have a big glass of milk and a slice of toast. That will stop your stomach from aching and cut the taste of disinfectant in your mouth," she advises. "And try getting some sleep. You've got a big day tomorrow." The door closes.

* * *

Later that day, I call Andy from my new Cork apartment to share last night's near-death experience and that Ivan, the Man with a Van, is due to arrive at his house around 2 p.m. to collect my boxes.

"I sent you a little something to thank you for everything you've done."

"You shouldn't have, Ams, although it is most welcome," he says about the case of wine that arrived yesterday. "I'm opening a bottle of Alberiño as we speak."

"Consider it a small token of appreciation."

Pop. Glug. Glug. I take that as a "yes".

"It was perfect timing, if you could call it that. It's not as if I had any visitors staying over. Speaking of visitors, we'll hopefully see you in Cork soon, assuming you don't move back to Dublin again or ingest something stronger than bottle steriliser. Only messing."

"Once was enough," I sigh. "I'm ready to settle back into my old life. I just hope I can pick up where I left off."

"I know starting over again is hard, Ams, but it beats standing still. We'll have plenty of that over the next few months of quarantine."

"Perfect timing, as you say."

Andy is right. Now happily ensconced in my new-ish digs, it's back to staying at home: no visiting, no travelling outside a five-kilometre radius, and if this continues longer than the first wave, a niggling question mark over making ends meet. Although the fashion industry is top-heavy with terms such as 'must have' and 'need now', no one is saving lives with hemlines. Frontline workers, we are not. I have no cause to complain as I remain safely indoors, but I worry about the future, especially as a single freelancer. Truth be told, my finances could use a triage. I don't have much to show for myself since the start of the pandemic other than a banjaxed shoulder from that photo shoot in September. Not that I do myself any favours. The lift in my apartment block is neither six feet wide nor long. Unless I 'must have' or 'need now' a contact tracing alert from the COVID-19 tracker app or the Delta variant as a housewarming present, I'll be ferrying my worldly belongings from the moving van solo.

Nothing a hot water bottle and Sunday on the sofa won't fix. My luck *is* turning for the better, after all. Finding an apartment in my old building during a global pandemic, not to mention Mercury Retrograde – those are some good odds. The analgesic rush of adrenaline, in the meantime, is a bonus. It's one small hurdle before a big new start. Well, *new-ish*.

* * *

November 2020

I'm lying on my bed in pain, wishing for something stronger than aspirin or ibuprofen. The once dull ache in my shoulder pinches, stabs and throbs. I can't sleep on my right side. I can't even lift my arm above my head without crying in agony. I try taking a shower but can't unclasp my bra. Nope. Not today, Satan. Instead, I look at the ceiling wondering, *Do I cut it off or wash with it on?* When I remember how much I paid for the death trap, I decide on the latter. It's moisture-wicking, after all.

Then it happens. Twitch. A small involuntary movement in my fingers. Like the flutter of a butterfly's wings. Nearly imperceptible. Except it isn't. It's noticeable. *I notice it.* No longer stymied by distractions and moving to-do lists, I can feel its amplitude increase. Day by day, I watch it grow until it becomes a steady shake, undulating with a wavelike rhythm. It's strange. What feels like a nervous jitter has no provenance, no narrative arc, no explanation. It just appears. Out of nowhere. Idiopathic. My mind naturally wanders and finds a cul-de-sac of conclusions courtesy of Google.

"Hand tremors can be a symptom of Parkinson's disease (PD), multiple sclerosis (MS), or dystonia. They can also occur following a stroke or traumatic brain injury. However, essential tremors are one of the most common causes of hand tremors and can occur without any other neurological signs," according to *Medical News Today*.

Slightly concerned and unable to see my GP, I call Margaret for a second opinion. She may be a numbers gal, but she's also a self-titled 'Mother Hen' and the boss of us sisters, like it or not.

"I'm no medic," she confesses, "but I think we're dealing with a trapped nerve."

That doesn't sound too bad, I think to myself.

"From what I know, it involves an operation and significant downtime – about four to six weeks."

After months of what passes as employment, the short-term prospect of being laid up and laid off sends me into a mini spiral.

"Please, Ams, don't stress about it," she insists. "The operation is incredibly painful but easy to bounce back from. If the pain continues to escalate, it may need immediate attention. Think of it this way: if it's affecting your work and your life, six weeks is a small trade-off." My sister, the shit-sandwich specialist. Her ability to layer bad news with just enough of the good to make it palatable never ceases to amaze me.

Before I hang up, she makes me promise to see my GP when the country reopens, which seems like the punchline of a bad joke. I need to remind myself that what feels like an eternity is only my mind interpreting time like I did as a child – slowly and with little to do. So, I turn my routines into rituals: I put on makeup every morning, I sit at the kitchen table for a cooked meal, I get some fresh air and tell myself, *Nothing lasts forever*.

Soon, it will be the holiday season, and if COVID numbers stay low, a sense of normality might return. Going somewhere besides the supermarket would be a treat. The last time I met friends was standing outside the local corner shop in the rain, our hands wrapped around lukewarm coffee, sharing nothing new from six feet apart. For Christmas this year, I'd prefer to catch a single silver fox than a novel virus, but I'll settle for a low R-value, covered outdoor seating and some decent small talk. I'm keeping my expectations low and hopes high. Let's see what happens.

December 2020

As if by the power of a Christmas miracle, the government announces a return to Level 2 restrictions. I'm spending Christmas week with my sister Patricia and her family in Galway, as is our tradition. Rather than risk me becoming a super-spreader on a three-hour coach journey, she drives to Cork to collect me. Also, I can't drive. Correction: I can hill start, weirdly enough, but I have no depth perception or concept of speed. This means I think every vehicle going in the opposite direction is about to mow me down, even though I just ran three red lights.

You see, a lifetime ago, I passed my driver's theory test, took the requisite lessons and applied for my learner's permit. However, my instructor politely advised me to practise in a parking lot before ever going on the road – if at all. Living mainly in cities, I never needed a car until I moved to the Cork suburbs. With my apartment only five kilometres outside the centre of town, buses and cabs are my primary means of getting around. Thus, I am subject to the vagaries of Cork Mean Time (CMT), where timetables and estimated arrivals are mostly for entertainment, and traffic is a given. So are no-shows and ghosting. Once familiar with an empirical understanding of CMT, walking doesn't seem so bad. Unless it's raining. And, boy, does it ever.

Forty-seven, single, still rents, can't drive: I can safely say I'm questioning my life choices. Not for long, though, as

Patricia has a knack for keeping me focused on the here and now and, more importantly, what's ahead. She's a Capricorn, which makes her bone practical. She's also a fraternal twin to my sister Maureen, which makes her self-reliant but super social. I could live at the top of Brow Head and she'd visit me. No questions asked. Correction: she'd probably stop for a coffee at Crookhaven and advise me this is not the hill on which she intends to die, proverbially or otherwise. Hey, everyone has their limits.

When she arrives at my apartment, it feels like Christmas has come early. "I haven't seen you since July!" I shriek as I hug her. We exchange a rapid-fire of words, thoughts, sidebars, gossip and giddiness before she does what she does best. Notice.

"Have you called your doctor yet about that tremor?

"Are you still having trouble sleeping?

"You should tell her about your restless legs, too. They might be related."

Aside from her honesty, Patricia is blessed with eyes in the back of her head and a nose that can detect if you ate garlic three days ago. She also point-blank knows when someone is lying. I frequently tell her she should get a side hustle with the police force, extracting confessions and sniffing out contraband. *She's that good.* So, when she points out something that has escaped my attention or has yet to present itself as a problem, I listen.

"No, to all the above," I admit. "But I'm on it. I solemnly pinkie swear."

"I'm only saying this because it's unusual for you. Of all people!" she implores, touching the door's wood panelling twice for luck. I pat my head jokingly in response.

"You're the least athletic of us five but the healthiest."

She's right. Six foot tall, I am the physical equivalent of 'failure to launch'. I flunked pre-school swimming lessons, struggled to run in elementary school and kept the bench warm for my secondary school basketball team. When God was doling out sporting genes, I was, most likely, commandeering the style and deportment queue. So, not an athlete. Nope. Not even close. I might get my height from my dad, but my health comes from my mom. She always says, "If it weren't for my side of the family, you girls wouldn't stand a chance." A bit harsh, but she has a point.

Her clan hails from Inishbofin, an island eight kilometres off the Connemara coast on the west of Ireland. Maybe it's the sea air or the Spanish-Norman gene pool, but they're a hearty bunch. Mom is robust, not unlike her mother, my Nana, who lived until she was almost 102. Dad, on the other hand, died at age 37 from a brain haemorrhage brought on by HHT (hereditary hemorrhagic telangiectasia), a rare vascular disorder which presents as red spots on the body that burst and bleed unprompted or when provoked. Both my sisters Margaret and Catherine have the condition, while my twin sisters struggle with asthma. Me? I only go to the doctor for routine check-ups. Somewhere in my mind, I know this is dumb luck.

"The universe doesn't give out free passes," I tell Patricia. "If you hear about someone getting knocked down by the 220 bus from Carrigaline, that'll be me."

"If that's the case," she teases, "be sure you're wearing clean knickers. While I'm here, show me where you keep your hair dye. Your greys are starting to show."

January 2021

Adapt. Pivot. Overcome. Such is the messaging that defines the third wave of COVID-19 and another stint of Level 5 lockdown restrictions. The government gives it a special touch by making Christmas Eve the day the country closes shop – just before Santa arrives. Nice one, lads. I suppose we should be grateful for the bit of leeway to travel back home after the turkey dinner. That is, of course, assuming you don't get a close contact alert on the COVID-19 app, like me. Happy New-ish Year! But how? I'm as good as monastic! After some pandemic maths and geotagging on my phone, I deduce the source was either the girl in the adjacent aisle on the coach back to Cork city or the taxi driver I hailed from the final stop on MacCurtain Street. Either way, I'm self-isolating. Not that it matters, as no one is going anywhere and it is now snowing. With time on my side (lots of time) and plenty of space to call my own, I brainstorm ways to keep relevant. Perching my laptop on the solid granite table, I remind myself I can do this: a bit of self-belief to oil the creative cogs.

Back in the day, I would fly to Paris and London this time of year to report on next season's collections, running from show to show and filing daily news copy, whether in a nearby cafe or backstage on a vacant stairwell. Then I would work through the night on additional fashion features, cursing the crappy Wi-Fi in my not-so-fancy hotel room and preparing a strategy for the next day's hustle. With show invitations from big fashion labels glaringly absent, I quickly learned how to work my angles as a persona non grata. Typically, this involved waiting for guests to find their seats before politely asking the nearest clipboard if I could stand and watch. Often, my request was accommodated as there were always a few VIPs who were no-shows. No one wants a patchy front row, especially a panicked production assistant who demands that you find a seat as soon as possible. Don't mind if I do. Sometimes it pays to be adaptable.

And so, mid-pandemic, I jockey for the elusive front row seat of ideas along with the rest of the world, vying for likes and comments, ready to sell a course or a widget. So, I order my ring light and lapel microphone from Amazon and prepare to join the popularity contest again. Although social media allows us the luxury of making a first impression twice, the measurement of success is in impressions – plural. This is going to be a slog. I can feel it already.

* * *

Not a lot changes over the next few weeks besides an increase in pandemic fatigue. No one is shopping. No one cares about what they are wearing. Our minds are focused on the seesaw of uncertainty that surrounds us. Like a sand artist on a windy day, I develop new ideas, only to wipe the slate clean. Instead, I busy myself hosting Instagram Live interviews with various fashion figures and advising people how to create wardrobe wellness with my closet decluttering tips. In doing so, I cultivate coping strategies to deal with this tremor. Its temperament is smooth and understated, but its velocity increases daily, which gives me pause but doesn't derail me.

It's all about the clever art of disguise, you see, learning what to conceal and reveal: something that comes second nature to me as a stylist. When recording any fashion content, I usually stand with my left hand facing the camera and my right resting on a prop such as a clothing rail. Similarly, I'll clasp my hands together to stem the vibration, tuck them under my arms like a bouncer, or adopt the Wonder Woman stance, hands on hips. My default pose is the air traffic controller. The way I see it, if I remain in a constant state of movement, it's guaranteed to keep one set of variables under control while I deal with the technical snafus of live recording. Plus, who can spot my hand shaking when my arm is doing an interpretive dance? Now, all

I need to do is get the disaster that passes for my hair to comply with some gel and root concealer. Grey by at least two fingers wide, my natural hairline resembles the road markings painted by the county council for vehicle access. At this rate, you could fit a Ford Fiesta on that regrowth no bother. Adapting, yes. Pivoting, maybe. Overcoming? That remains to be seen.

February 2021

I'm making pancakes, the American kind: thick and fluffy, begging for maple syrup. Outside the wind chill makes the temperature real-feel minus ten. Plus, there's that Irish special: sideways rain. I pour the last of the batter onto the frying pan, lowering the heat so it doesn't burn – and wait. I'm getting used to that. In about four minutes it will join the others stacked on the warming plate for no one to eat. I don't have much of an appetite, but I am a sucker for tradition, it being Pancake Tuesday and all. Besides, it gives me something to do other than wait for the waiting to end. The ennui is such that at the end of every day, I celebrate the things I achieve, however routine: getting out of bed, blowing my hair dry, making soup, filing my fashion column, developing a new pitch. Small wins.

As the mixture cooks, I siphon through the stack of letters and junk mail on top of the coffee machine. A postcard escapes from between two envelopes into my free hand, avoiding a sticky landing. It reads:

Happy Alternative Valentine's Day
Sending you love and good vibes in the universe to counteract the terrible effects of Mercury Retrograde (and the pandemic!).

Stay strong, soon we'll have COVID in the back mirror and will be able to meet up again, laugh about this and pour ourselves another glass of wine.
Lots of love,
Neil

Of course it is. Who else would it be? My heart and eyes fill up. Neil and I go way back. We met in 1998 after my then-flatmate introduced us. How could I forget? I wore purple spike-heeled snakeskin boots and took him clubbing, then insisted he carry my circus stilts while we walked home from Dublin's Leeson Street, with me wondering why no cabs would pick us up. Not much has changed. He is still patient and practical, while misplaced optimism is apt to render me barefoot.

Flipping the last pancake, I give him a quick call, thanking him for the card. "Solitary confinement is not a good look for me. I don't know how much more of it I can take."

"Have you seen Julie at all?" he asks. Julie is my neighbour and dear college friend whose shoes Neil has also carried.

"Yesterday, in fact," I say. "She's the only human I've spoken to face-to-face since I got back after Christmas. We sat on the wall outside of Centra and talked about the weather. Very Irish, I know. Then it started to rain. No surprises there."

"I know you're doing your bit on Insta, but staying connected in person with the likes of Julie, even outside on a wall in the rain, is super important." Neil senses my weariness. "It won't be long though, Ams. Numbers are steadily going down. Hang in there. How's your hand?"

I lift it to the overhead oven light. "It needs to be seen soon; the shake is worsening. That said, I did an awesome job with these pancakes."

Deflecting our conversation away from my messy emotions, I wrap things up, promising to talk later in the week. Considering how much the two of us chat and the forward-facing nature of my job, I'm lonely and most likely depressed. This I keep under wraps, not wanting to be a burden. I don't answer calls as often, preferring to respond by text or voice note. When I do talk, conversations are short and sweet. I turn inwards and keep others at an emotional distance. I'm my own worst enemy. Truth be told, I miss Margaret. Don't get me wrong, I love my own company, but I love it by choice. There is no choice with a pandemic. Alone is alone.

March 2021

As quarantine measures start to lift, public service announcements play on the radio, encouraging people to visit their GP for non-COVID-related health concerns. I'm ecstatic. Face time, but with actual faces – real people! More importantly, *answers*.

Several days later, I'm at my local medical centre, sharing the trajectory of my shoulder and tremor concerns under a three-ply mask with my GP. We discuss the likelihood of a rotator cuff or labral injury and possibilities outside of a trapped nerve, such as Parkinson's and essential tremor. While I'm there, I ask for a hormonal blood panel to get to the bottom of my petulant periods, a feat of bravery which involves me squeamishly looking away while she prepares the needle. After filling and labelling the test tubes, she writes me an MRI referral for my shoulder – the first of three in a search for answers. The next nine months are a waiting game. Because of the pressure placed on our health service by the pandemic, delays with clinic scans, hospital operations and consultant appointments are standard, if not expected. Being the youngest of five, I'm used to waiting my turn: last in the queue, as it were. In the interim, I apply for an online training course in radio writing and presenting to keep myself busy. Pivoting and all that. Well, it can't hurt.

June 2021

It's official. The world is finally reopening, or 'emerging' as the media calls it. Soon, we'll have a before and after. In the meantime, we occupy that liminal space: a vaccine, a haircut and a few visitors, but other than that, no sudden movements. Like a mole woman released from an underground bunker, I am sadly happy to be free. It's been so long that I don't know how to be anything else but inside.

I think back to an Instagram Live interview I hosted the month previous with the iconic drag queen Veda Lady. During our chat, we reminisced about a fashion spread for the *Sunday Times Style* in which she taught me how to make an entrance for the party season. The main image spoke volumes: me in a leather bondage dress with a metal neckpiece and *Game of Thrones*-style fake fur, trying to stifle the giggles as a spiky-haired Veda purred into my ear.

After months of self-isolating, I wonder if I can channel that same entrance-making energy to join life on the outside again, warrior queen cosplay aside. That fearlessness is inside me, somewhere. I know it is. The question is, where? In the meantime, I maintain the status quo and do what I do best: small indoor gatherings, ideally me and one other person – maybe two. Thanks to lockdown, I can add 'culinary amateur' to my bragging rights. That is, assuming there is no main course: starters, desserts, snacks, side dishes and sauces are my wheelhouse. Show me a chicken or a turkey and we may as well call emergency services because someone is getting salmonella. Luckily for my sister Catherine, Italian orzo and bean soup are on the menu, along with toasted sourdough bread and homemade hummus. The National Centre for HHT is located at Cork's Mercy University Hospital, so she's stopping by for a quick visit after her annual check-up.

A former New York police officer, Catherine now runs an artisan weaving business on Inishbofin. Married to the local postman, together they raise sheep and, at one stage, had a very affable donkey called Darwin. I tell you, this girl is a living, breathing Maeve Binchy novel. The day she rocks up in a lilac bus, I won't be surprised. Here's the thing about our Kate. Although her life reads like fiction, her manner is matter of fact. She doesn't deal with nuances or shades of grey, which makes her a perfect messenger for this next exchange.

After we eat and chew the fat, I show her around the apartment as it's her first time visiting me since my move back to Cork. Typically, we don't spend a lot of time together and can be more familial than familiar. While gesticulating mid-flow about something of little importance, my tremor becomes active. Without thinking, it takes refuge inside my trouser pocket as I prattle on about my bedroom slide robes. Kate looks straight at me and reads me my Miranda rights with her hazel eyes.

"You know, you don't have to hide."

As moments of vulnerability go, this is intense. I feel seen and laid bare all at once. Tears run down my face. She's right. I'm not being open with her. Instead, I hide behind niceties and small talk, choosing highlights and headlines over deep dives about what is going on in my life. The stiffness, the tremor, the bouts of insomnia – these might all wind up to be nothing, but what if they're something? What then?

Silence.

"It's getting worse, Kate . . ." I use my left hand to wipe my wet cheeks. "And the shoulder MRI didn't bring up anything unusual. I'm just so—"

Stuck on pause, she meets me halfway.

"—fed up, I know. Even more reason to visit your friends or go to Galway to see Patricia now that we can travel again," she suggests. "Besides, Rosie is therapy on four legs."

Rosie is Patricia's pug and beloved fur baby. An afternoon of zoomies, tug-of-war and belly rubs with her ladyship is like a shot of serotonin.

"You need your people. Don't forget that."

And I don't. This is the most important advice I'll ever hear.

July 2021

You know you're in Cork when you find a wall of Tanora in Tesco. But what I'm hunting for is a handheld fan – the heatwave equivalent of toilet paper at the start of the pandemic. The forecast says 'warm and breezy', but my hormonal body is convinced we're heading to Burning Man, not my brother-in-law's fiftieth. He and my sister Patricia and a couple of their friends are celebrating with a Cork staycation, so I'm meeting them later that evening for a drink at my local bar-restaurant. There's no joy on the handheld fan, so I grab a bottle of orange fizz from the wall. This will have to do.

Later that evening, I arrive at the outdoor seating area reserved for the party and Patricia waves me over. I'm wearing a short-sleeved Breton top and cropped trousers, but I may as well be wearing a down-filled sleeping bag wrapped in cling film. Although pints and Pornstar Martinis are on the go, a glass of chilled white wine finds its way to me. I get chatting with my sister and Brendan, my brother-in-law's best friend, about everything and nothing as beads of sweat multiply on my upper lip. Well-versed in the art of concealment, I pull a Princess Diana stealth move. Covering my mouth while coyly laughing at someone's joke, I buy enough time to wipe away the offending perspiration. It keeps happening. Patricia, true to form, clocks it straight away. She gives me the eye flash, which is code for "It's time to visit the ladies' room". Before I can excuse myself, I feel rivulets running down the side of my cheek and into the crook of my neck.

"I'm sorry, Brendan," I say, grabbing the nearest napkin to swab my face. "I'm not harbouring state secrets. It's just peri-menopause."

Being a gentleman, Brendan listens as I rant about persistent insomnia and bio-identical hormones. In retrospect, I may have scarred the poor guy, but social protocol gets the short shrift when conversation skills go to pasture. I do, however, keep the egregious details to myself, namely erratic periods (every 7 to 17 days), regular night sweats and significant hair loss. I shed so much it's as if a tiny hedgehog manifests in the drain after each shower.

This concerns me as much as my tremor, which now presents as a pronounced jerking movement from my hand to my shoulder. I excuse myself to use the bathroom. When I return, Patricia gives me that look. It's a precursor to another honesty sound bath. I have no choice but to bask in the well-intended questioning and honour it as coming from a place of love. Plus, she's always spot on, so who am I to argue? She lowers her voice and leans in, creating a buffer of chestnut brown curls between us and the rest of the group.

"Do you know your right foot drags when you walk?
"Your right arm is jerking up to your shoulder now.
"Blink, Annmarie. You're doing that staring thing again. It's freaking me out!"

I blink. Then I laugh. Don't ask me how, but I have a recently acquired tic where I zone out for a second too long. My eyes fixate on nothing in particular. My brain disengages for a beat. It's like being held hostage by a synaptic lapse. Still convinced an undetected trapped nerve is the culprit, despite evidence to the contrary, I wait patiently for the results of the second MRI to validate my unprofessional opinion.

September 2021

What a difference a year makes – or doesn't, depending on how you look at it. Twelve months, three physio sessions, two MRIs, one orthopaedic consultant and a set of would-be symptoms later, I'm older but still none the wiser. To think that a sore shoulder could cause this much fuss. While we scratch our heads, I'm figuring out how to finesse my fine motor skills into completing essential tasks so that I can get paid.

Now that people are beginning to shop again, I am creating online seminars about the future of workwear for corporates heading back to the office. The rigid fingers on my right hand are increasingly non-compliant, either refusing to move or tapping uncontrollably. Periodically, I stop and massage my hands until they regain flexibility. Sometimes they don't. That's why I'm learning to type left-handed. My fingers usually move like those of a pianist: fast and fluid, often outperforming the pace of my thoughts. Assignments that would take two days now take three – time I can ill afford to lose. God, I need some answers. And before I know it, my phone rings.

It's not God, but close enough. It's my GP with the all-clear on my neck and spine MRI. Although great news, it still doesn't shed any light on the nature of my tremor, so she organises another referral – this time for a brain scan to make sure there is nothing more serious at play. She also puts me on the waiting list for a neurologist. Despite having personal health insurance, I simply don't have the resources to go private. The €200 I pay the osteopathic consultant, confirming my shoulder scan results, pushes my credit card to its limit. Given the considerable delay of the past two MRIs, my next appointment could take a while. At least this way I'll be in the system. Plus, as you know, I am a Zen master in the art of waiting.

I then remember the videos I recorded of my tremor during the summer; she asks me to email them to her. Having a visual like a video to share with a neurologist is always useful and might prove helpful in getting me seen earlier. It's no guarantee, but worth a shot. The waiting game continues.

October 2021

Just act like nothing happened. My eyes scan for witnesses as I high-speed reverse my faceplant. *Nothing to see here, folks.* In the detergent aisle, there's a mom with two screaming kids and a man wearing what looks like a hazmat helmet – both too preoccupied to notice me tripping over my own two feet. So much for Scandi chic. Every time I wear these damn sneakers, I add insult to personal injury claim. Today is one of those days. I gather my washing powder and TV snacks off the floor and hobble over to the till.

Fashion victim leanings aside, something is wrong. My symptoms are taking a sinister turn. Maybe I'm overthinking it or maybe I just need a pair of sneakers that aren't out to kill me;

either way, I need to do something. My right leg visibly drags. The slowness is scary – that feeling of being weighed down by an invisible magnet, my lengthy strides contracting to a fraction of their usual speed. It doesn't stack up. I may not be athletic, but my long limbs always stand me in good stead.

According to urban legend, I once pushed a stalled taxi during a snowstorm in high heels, which did their civic duty as crampons. Until recently, I was also able to wrap my legs around my arms and walk on my hands (everyone needs a party piece). But now . . .

What is happening? Am I being demonically possessed? I tap my phone to discover it won't accept my Google Pay. Something weird is afoot. *No kidding*, I think to myself. With no cash and my debit card in the apartment, I walk home from the shop empty-handed.

Late that evening, with it being Halloween, I'm bingeing season four of the sci-fi horror series *Stranger Things*, albeit with no snacks. In the first episode, Vecna – a sentient humanoid with an axe to grind – mysteriously murders two high school students. Forcing the victims into a levitating trance, he brutally snaps and pulls apart their bones like they're a side order of chicken wings, opening a small gate to an alternate dimension known as the Upside Down. What has reportedly terrified fans of the franchise looks like an average Saturday night in my world. Thursday and Friday, too, if you count last week.

The casual nighttime foot cramps I mistakenly blame on low magnesium now feel malicious. The stiffness and spasms give me no warning, catching me on the hop (pun intended) as my right foot contorts, arch levitating and toes separating like they are about to break. Such is the pain that it only dissipates after many expletives, much jumping around and a lot of crying. Welcome to my personal Upside Down.

Given the weird nocturnal activity, I'm happy, if not relieved, to be single. Besides, I can't envisage anyone sticking around for long with the likelihood of diabolic visitations. It's a bit of a mood-killer. Not to mention my restless legs, which used to only happen before my monthly cycle and are now a nightly occurrence. Considering I hate dancing, it's ironic that I'm forced into regular renditions of *Riverdance* right before I nod off. Assuming I do fall asleep, the real problem is staying that way. Awake most nights, I feel as if I'm in an altered state of consciousness. I'd venture as far as to say, "I'm haunted" – only in Cork, the phrase has a different meaning. With my brain scan pending, I might have too much time to think, but whatever is happening to my body is giving me plenty of reason to ruminate. Then it hits me. It's not an MRI, magnesium, a massage or even a new pair of sneakers that I need. It's a bloody exorcist.

November 2021

Knock, knock. I'm visiting my first closet decluttering client in almost two years. For the record, my bank account is very excited.

"Arlene?"

"Hi. Come on in. You found us," she delights.

"So sorry about earlier. My Google Maps must need updating." This is a white lie. My sense of direction is remedial at best. Combine this with a petulant tremor and the joys of predictive text for best results.

A cup of tea is on offer, biscuits if I like, which I politely decline, suggesting we get a start on what promises to be a busy day. Besides, I can't risk the caffeine in case I get jittery. So far, so good.

"I took your advice: quiet house and comfy clothes," she says, pointing to her denim shirt and joggers. "The hubby has the dog and the kids for the next few hours."

Inside the bedroom are piles of clothes stacked neatly on the mattress, shoes line the wall and a roll of black sacks sit on top of the underwear drawer. "These are items I need help styling," she shows me, "and those are ones I'm not sure about keeping. I thought it might make it easier to see them laid out."

"So many people clean and get rid of things before I come, which sort of defeats the purpose," I confide, "so, thank you for doing this. It's so important to see a person's real wardrobe as it is."

"Well, as I mentioned in the questionnaire you sent me, gaining the COVID stone has limited what I can wear and, to be honest, put a dent in my confidence. I also have psoriasis, which flares up with stress, so . . ."

"Nothing we can't sort out," I reassure her, appreciative that she's invited me into her personal space. We address what's on the bed and before long are making inroads on her walk-in wardrobe. I can feel my tremor acting up here and there. I'm pretty sure she notices. I try my arsenal of poses, which just makes me look fidgety and a bit odd, standing like Wonder Woman amidst overfed plastic bags. To distract from the shaking, I make frequent trips in and out of the closet. The tremor is getting jerky, and I'm getting tired. I think about what Kate said. It's time to come clean. There's nothing to hide.

"About this," I say, pointing to my hand. "I've acquired a weird shake since lockdown. Nothing major. It just gets pesky now and again. I wanted to let you know in case you thought I was partying last night."

She gives a nonchalant "No bother," insisting, "Everyone's got something, don't they?"

I agree. *Whatever 'something' is.*

December 2021

Something's missing. Christmas feels flat. My tree is the first to go up each November: a ten-foot pine monolith with enough gewgaws to cancel quiet luxury. And for what? So that the yuletide spirit can ghost me. This can't happen. I'm Santa's cheerleader, a festive fundamentalist, goodwill's self-appointed hunter. 'Tis my season but where's the jolly?

To be honest, this all makes me very nervous. As a child, uncertainty was the bearer of bad tidings and familiar enough to breed contempt. Opening my presents on Christmas morning in 1977, I remember feeling like someone sucked the magic out of the room. There was an absence I couldn't describe, but a detail I'll never forget – the packages were covered in pastel tissue paper. These weren't from Santa. My father's colleagues in the police department delivered them – candy-coloured condolences from the 42nd Precinct. That I knew. Even as a kid, they felt like a consolation prize, only I wasn't sure what I had lost.

I have a similar feeling today, though there are no pastels in sight. The memory makes me hold my breath. *Think positively. You had your brain scan last Wednesday, so the results will be back soon,* I tell myself. No more waiting. Of that, I am certain. It's time for something different. To keep the magic alive and the absence at bay, I volunteer to present a radio slot for the festive period on Christmas FM Classical. I see it as a chance to hone my fledgling skills, support their charity partner and sustain that feel-good feeling. Each week, I pre-record my three-hour show from home, crafting links from my DIY bedroom studio, which I soundproof with blankets and throw pillows.

I'm Annmarie O'Connor. I'll be with you until six this evening. It's just gone three o'clock. You're very welcome wherever you're listening. Coming up, we have continuous classical and carols, including Joel Cohen's "Joy to The World" and the Choir of Winchester Cathedral performing "Lullaby My Jesus".

Someone once told me I have the kind of voice that breaks the news when you've got three weeks to live. An unusual compliment, perhaps, but I appreciated the sentiment. Although my speaking style is easy on the ear, listening back to my song links, it has noticeably softened. In the interests of clarity, I record the links twice, projecting more consciously into the microphone. Coming from a talkative family where airtime is precious, she who speaks loudest gets heard. Being audible is never a concern. I simply adjust my volume button where necessary. As red flags go, this is pink at best; something worth noting but not worth worrying about, or so I think.

What occupies my attention most is my tremor: the wilful toddler who is testing my last nerve with its bratty behaviour. Each time I save a recorded link, my fingers remain rigid. Then my hand jerks, causing me to cut the audio in the wrong spot or worse, delete it. It is messing with my magic-making MO. As for sending Christmas cards? My handwriting, now small and cramped, means my season's greetings look more like ransom notes. Not exactly festive.

The more I try to fill the absence, the more my symptoms seem to intensify. One morning, I nearly impale myself putting on earrings and I tap out in a fight to the death with a set of false lashes. Applying mascara is next to impossible, which, in my opinion, should be a hate crime. I always joke that vanity will be the death of me (usually when wearing a pair of five-inch spike heels), but today, it's no laughing matter.

More worryingly, my right hand is beginning to curl inwards, challenging me to brush my teeth without impaling my gums or open a bag of coffee without sending espresso across the kitchen. As low points go, struggling to get my caffeine fix sounds pedestrian, but it gets my attention. The things I take for granted – the everyday bliss-bringers, the magic – are being sucked out of the room. It's like watching my identity being stolen in slow motion. Enough is enough.

Right on cue, the phone rings. It's my GP confirming the all-clear on my brain scan results. I'm relieved and dissatisfied in equal measure. So is she, especially when I share the recent escalation in my symptoms: the jerking, the shaking, the rigidity. I need to see a neurologist. With the waiting lists being what they are, she arranges for me to attend Cork University Hospital's (CUH) acute medical unit the next day for further tests. After nine months of waiting, I might just get an answer.

CHAPTER TWO
Diagnosis
The news

December 16, 2021

I ARRIVE AT CUH shortly before 9 a.m., armed with my Kindle, a phone recharger and hopes of clarity. After signing in, I find a plastic chair in an almost empty row. The weather on the wall-sprung TV reveals it's unseasonably warm for the time of year, a fact confirmed by my bare ankles. A woman seated in front of me looks unbothered by tulips in December. So does the man to the left of her. This could be a long day. I take it as a cue to start reading *Less Is Lost* – a road trip adventure about a writer who tries to escape his problems after a financial crisis and the death of an old lover. I admit, renting a van and hitting the open road holds a certain appeal, but I would be too anxious for it to be worth the effort. Life, in the end, always catches up with you. Plus, what do you pack?

I don't get very far with the misadventures of my antihero. Most of my day is spent with various medical staff who make their determinations before I meet with a neurologist. First, the nurse takes my vitals and bloodwork. Then, I chat periodically with different doctors about my medical history and the origin story of my symptoms. Around lunch, an orderly comes by with a cart of chicken and stuffing sandwiches, biscuits and tea.

Shortly before 4 p.m., I meet the consultant neurologist, who introduces himself as Dr Sweeney. After a briefing and another chat about my health odyssey, we begin a series of physical tests, some of which include rapid finger and toe-tapping, walking heel-to-toe and in a straight line, standing up from a chair with my arms crossed at the chest, hands at rest and then moving and producing a handwriting sample. These, I would soon discover, assess slowness, rigidity, tremor, gait and balance abnormalities – the hallmarks of a certain degenerative brain disorder. After what feels like 20 minutes and a final discussion with his colleague, he delivers his diagnosis. I have early-onset Parkinson's disease. Absolute. Affirmative. Crystal clear.

The words don't penetrate. They can't. Even the truth takes time. Instead, I accept the news like a third-party proxy – dispassionate and attentive. Still standing from our battery of tests, he invites me to sit down. Here it gets hazy, but I do recall what would be the first of many chats about the disease.

I have Parkinson's? Surely there's been a mistake. This can't actually be happening.

Sure, I'd heard of actor Michael J. Fox, who was diagnosed at age 29, and boxer Mohammed Ali, who was diagnosed at age 42, but they must be the exceptions to the rule, right? Wrong. Here's what I now know.

Parkinson's disease (also known as Parkinson's or PD) is a chronic, progressive, neurodegenerative disorder affecting the levels of dopamine in the brain. Currently, there is no cure. Dopamine is one of the brain's many chemical messengers. You may know it as the 'reward' drug: the pay-off you get from feel-good activities like sex, shopping or smelling cookies.

Aside from delivering pleasure, it is also responsible for controlling movement, mood and motivation, amongst other crucial functions.

In people with Parkinson's, roughly 60 to 80 per cent of nerve cells that produce dopamine have died by the time symptoms appear, of which there are over 40, both motor and non-motor related. The result? Life-limiting problems from losing the ability to speak, smell, swallow or emote to postural instability, balance issues and falls, not to mention tremors and, in later stages of the disease, having to rely on a caregiver. And all this time I thought dopamine simply drove me to impulse-buy and scroll too much on social media.

Dr Sweeney explains to me that as someone who is early- or young-onset (usually between the age of 21 and 50) and in the early stages of Parkinson's, the disease tends to be slow-moving, with motor symptoms typically affecting one side of the body.

For me, it's my right-hand side. When I look back, it all makes sense: the shaking, the slowness, the stiffness; things like my leg dragging, the foot spasms I now know as 'dystonia', and one which I never registered – a reduced arm swing when I walk.

As for my tremor, I am told that Parkinson's is typically 'resting'. In other words, it is active while my right hand is at rest. An essential tremor, on the other hand, is active when moving, like reaching for something from a shelf or pouring a cup of tea. Some people can have both.

The non-motor symptoms like insomnia, fatigue and anxiety, however, are sneakier and share similarities with other conditions, such as menopause or even a case of the pandemic blues. Yet, not once did I consider Parkinson's disease. Despite being a hot contender to a trapped nerve (although that was ruled out by my first MRI) and essential tremor, I never thought to dig deeper. I never thought it could happen to me.

To an extent, I was right. Of the estimated 10 million people with Parkinson's globally, there are only 18,000 living in Ireland, roughly 40 per cent of whom are female. Apply this math to the 10 per cent of people classified as early-onset in our country and the numbers are smaller still.

To make things more niche, of Parkinson's 40-plus symptoms, no two people have the same combination. I suppose that's why people refer to it as the 'boutique disease'. If that's the case, mine's a limited-edition exclusive. I won't lie: a vintage Hermès Kelly bag would have been preferable. I wonder does the universe take returns? Levity may help, but it doesn't erase the reality of a long-term illness. Compassionate and reassuring, Dr Sweeney acknowledges its impact on someone with dreams and ambitions yet unfulfilled, let alone daily responsibilities. I think of my third book, now stalled at 25,000 words, the fashion features I write and the photo shoots I style – my bread and butter. He notices how I disguise my tremor under the crooks of my arms, in my pocket, hand over hand, stratagems which I unconsciously deployed in the past half hour. Side note: Patricia would be deeply satisfied with his acuity. Still puzzled, I ask him about the results of my recent scan.

"If I have Parkinson's, why was the brain scan clear?"

Seemingly, Parkinson's lives a few millimetres below what an MRI can see, and as there is no specific lab or imaging test for PD, diagnoses are clinical. Using a more sophisticated dopamine transporter scan (DaTscan) can rule out Parkinson's mimics and help a patient's peace of mind, but this is to support a diagnosis which is, I am told, affirmative.

I have Parkinson's. It just isn't landing.

Sensing my disbelief, Dr Sweeney mentions that if I decide to manage my condition with medication, I will get further confirmation in about the first week. Traditionally, Parkinson's symptoms are treated with a dopaminergic drug called levodopa, or L-dopa for short. Known as 'the gold standard', L-dopa works by being converted into dopamine in the brain. Only Parkinson's responds to this drug, so if things improve, I'll know like I know.

Aware that I will retain only a fraction of our conversation, he asks me to return to the CUH outpatient department the following week to discuss treatment options and the future in more detail. He also advises me to bring a second pair of ears to catch what escapes mine. Smart man.

I sign out of the unit and walk towards the hospital gates. *I have Parkinson's.* Those three words run through my head like a breaking news chyron. I don't know what to feel or how my life figures in all of this. Well, the bottom line is if my symptoms improve with medication, I can get back to being me, but with the trade-off of having a progressive, incurable brain disorder. Certainly not the news I was hoping for, but I tell myself it's something to work with.

Only it's not. Despite having the answers I need, I have no roadmap, no directions on the back of a packet, no what to do in case of an emergency. The absence revisits me like it did Christmas morning in 1977. I am unprepared. I am lost.

My mom rings. Still in a haze, I answer the call, pre-empting her usual, "Hello, dear. I hope I haven't caught you at a bad time."

"Mom, I have Parkinson's," I blurt. No hello. No nothing. Then it hits me . . .

"I don't know what to do."

Not a lot knocks my mother, who at age 35 became a widow with five children. Her life changed without her permission one not-so-average afternoon. An afternoon when my dad screamed in pain. An afternoon where he was rushed to hospital and put on machines that would keep him alive, machines that would dry the blood from his lungs and stop him from choking. An afternoon where his brain was dead and hope wasn't far behind. An afternoon where my mother knew like she knew. He wasn't coming back. Three weeks later, he died.

She told me once that she had a feeling it was too good to be true – a loving marriage, a wonderful husband. She was always waiting for the other shoe to drop. And when it did, nothing quite prepared her for that knock, but nothing quite knocked her again.

"Dear, you'll carry on," she tells me with quiet certainty, "and you'll do it because you have to. That's all you can do."

We say our goodbyes as I step into the fading December light.

One foot in front of the other, I tell myself. Soon it will be dark.

* * *

I call a cab but I don't remember anything about the journey, aside from leaving messages for my sisters and a text for Julie, my neighbour and one of my closest friends, who is currently working from home.

Would you have time to call over this evening? I write. *Neurologist told me I have Parkinson's disease. Sorry to drop that on you. I still can't believe it. Xx*

Of course, she replies. *I will be over. Give me 15 mins. Xxx*

Unlocking the door to my apartment, I am relieved to be home. Shock doesn't often disarm me. Not in the moment, anyway.

Instead, I turn on the Christmas tree lights and ask my Google Assistant to play some festive tunes. Andy Williams croons about it being the most wonderful time of the year. *Debatable*, I think to myself, but hum along, regardless. Now comfortably dislocated from the heart of the news, its gravitas hangs outside of my psyche. Here, my inner monologue adopts a palliative yet practical tone.

At least they caught it early. I am young and healthy. My body will respond to medication. No more hiding my hands to stem the shaking and jerking. No more trying to write features while my rigid fingers stage a boycott. No more painful foot cramps when waking in the morning or insomnia from nightly restless legs. No more stiffness and slowness. My life will be manageable again.

The video monitor alerts me to someone at the door. It's Julie – two minutes early. She hugs me as if I just lost a family member. "I'm so sorry," she says. I can feel her pain for me. Reflexive empathy, they call it. I call it three decades of friendship. To say we have history is an understatement. We not only know where the bodies are buried, we both have a shovel.

A practical Taurean like myself, she pairs wine with her sympathy and hands me a bottle of well-needed Sauvignon Blanc. My kind of first responder. We chat as I pour us two medicinal glasses; she listens and I process. Like my sisters, she's seen my health depreciate in real time and knows that the course of my life has altered, despite being better for the diagnosis. The physical and emotional changes, the adjustments to my lifestyle, my career and my sense of self – all these things will happen sooner rather than later.

Some things, though, never change. We're still the fun-loving drama queens who met at university. The aspiring actor and the writer who moved to London together, working sensible jobs by day and serving beers in bars at night. We're the girls who minded each other, who learned from each other, who got by together and thrived together. We're definitely the girls who caused way too much devilment together. Now, as we get older, we have stories that make us laugh and memories that make us blush. Most of all, we have each other. You can't put a price on that.

I ask her to be my extra set of ears at next week's appointment.

"Of course, I'll take you wherever you need to go, Annie."

"I know, Jules."

She grabs my hand. I grab hers. Reflexive empathy.

One of Mozart's piano sonatas interrupts our *Thelma & Louise* moment. It's Margaret.

"Answer it, Annie." Julie motions towards my phone as she puts on her coat. "I have to get going, anyway."

Before I swipe up on the green icon, I know what's ahead of me. Upon receiving the news of my diagnosis, Mags will have pressed the proverbial emergency button and engaged her plan of action. Despite being a corporate director (to this day, I can never remember her job title), acts of service is her love language, especially in a crisis. Today, this involves running to Penneys to buy me pyjamas, stocking up on soup and informing me she's on a mercy mission to Cork.

"Mags, I'm not sick."

"But you have Parkinson's."

"I know. I've had it since last September, or at least that we know of."

"I can be there in three hours. Two and a half with no traffic."

"Don't be daft. You have friends arriving from Australia tomorrow."

"I'll cancel."

"Mags, I love you, but please stay put. I need to get some sleep and let this sink in before I figure out what happens next. I don't even know anything about the disease."

"I'll do some research. Give me an hour. I can—"

"Mags," I interrupt. "It's OK. I'll be OK. It's going to be OK. Please don't worry."

"It's my job to worry."

"No, it's not. It's your job to be a . . ."

"You still don't know what I do for a living, do you?"

"Not a clue. I just know you do it well."

"My phone is beside my bed. If you need anything at any time of the night, promise to call me."

"I promise. And Mags?"

"Yes."

"Thanks for the pyjamas."

December 17, 2021

Julie is away for the day at a family function with her husband and three kids. I promise to walk and feed her cocker spaniel, Joy, which gives me a focus and some well-needed exercise. Joy, too. She loves a good sniff: hedges, a grassy verge, my sneakers, lampposts – any and every random scent. Our favourite route is the boreen off Maryborough Hill, where I play fantasy real estate and Joy gets her country fix before we head back to the suburbs. On my way home from Julie's, my sister Maureen calls. She's Patricia's twin and is a bona fide Earth Mother. Colourful, caring and always chatty, she's not afraid to take up space and can fill a room with her hearty laugh. Where Patricia does minutiae, Maureen does broad brushstrokes. Most of all, she is unapologetically herself and has the boundaries to prove it. Overstep them and you'll soon get a rude awakening.

Once I hear her warm voice, I find a seat on the wall of the corner shop which, until recently, has been the centre of my social life.

"I didn't want to call you last night, so I just left a message. I knew you'd need some space."

"You're right. It was a lot to get my head around," I agree, adding that I had Julie for company and a good night's sleep. "Margaret rang."

"I know. I had a word with her."

"You did?"

"You know Mags, Ams. She's a good egg, but her default is crisis management. I think she forgets this is something you've been living with for over a year."

"She was about to come to Cork, Mo. I could practically hear the car keys rattling in her hand."

"She still thinks you might change your mind. I had to remind her this isn't her battle to fight and that you will tell us what you need and when you need it, in your own time."

On the surface, Maureen is a talker, but at heart, she's a listener. Her gift? Knowing that the greatest act of service is to give people what they need, not what *you* think they need. She also knows that behind my outgoing persona is a lesser-spotted introvert. I need time to myself: time to reflect, decompress, concentrate, make decisions. It's in retreat that I find rest – a place to allow my mind to unwind. Only then can I show up in the world fully and authentically. And when I don't? I people-please, keep the peace, let things slide. Needless to say, it never ends well.

"Look, Ams. This is your journey. You've got to be the one to set the agenda and decide what's best for you. Don't worry you'll offend us. You won't. Just be honest."

I think of the message I sent to the family group chat this morning – a seasoned spin-doctor massaging the narrative –

and I realise I need to be honest with myself first. Not only do I have the kind of voice that can break bad news, but I'm gullible enough to think it's not that bad.

After about 20 minutes, my bum cheeks are expressing their discomfort. I rock from side to side, but the stones are majority shareholders on this wall. "I better go," I groan, before standing up to smooth the bumpy imprints from the backs of my leggings.

"Any plans when you get home?"

"I'll probably do a few hours' research, compile questions for next week's outpatient appointment and decide what life on long-term medication looks like. You know, light weekend stuff."

"Promise me you'll never use the term *new normal*."

"It goes without saying."

We agree to catch up later in the week before both of us realise I'll be on my way to Galway for Christmas break by then. "Hey, before you hang up," Maureen asks, "can you do me a favour? Please ring Margaret and put her out of her misery. She's like a nurse on-call with those pyjamas in the back seat of her car."

December 21, 2021

I hate being late. This sentiment is being put to the test by the unfamiliar route to St Catherine's Convent – the CUH neurology outpatient unit. Remarkably, I'm the one giving Julie directions as the Google Assistant stages a silent protest. Even *she* thinks it's below her pay grade.

"Turn left onto Model Farm Road and continue straight before you turn left across from the pub on the right. Then take another right before taking the first left . . ."

Somehow, by the grace of God, we arrive.

With time to spare, Julie parks the car and I sign in at reception. Shortly after taking a seat in the waiting room, I hear my name being called by my consultant. As we exchange masked pleasantries and get seated in the office, I pull out my notebook and its list of questions. Julie raises an eyebrow in approval, impressed by my preparation. I feel like I'm at a job interview until it occurs to me that there's no right way of doing Parkinson's. No one is grading me. It's best if I keep that in mind.

Today, we revisit much of what we discussed during my diagnosis with more of a focus on how to make this work for me, Annmarie.

Here's the thing about Parkinson's. It's a tough pill to swallow. As someone with early-onset, the disease will likely develop slowly, but being incurable and progressive, it's guaranteed to play catch up.

This is one day at a time. Every person is different. Dr Sweeney has even treated a guy in his teens who is now older and living a happy and healthy life.

One foot in front of the other.

The question I need to consider is if I want to start medication or not. Bearing in mind that the drugs only treat the symptoms over time, and with habituation, dosages will need to be adjusted to sustain their desired effect. A lifetime dictated by timers, pillboxes and diaries. Can I handle it?

Of course, lifestyle also plays a crucial part. Things like a healthy diet, hydration, sleep hygiene and regular exercise can also improve wellbeing and exercise is known to slow down the progression of the disease. Individually or in tandem, neither option is a magic bullet, both having their pros and cons.

There's more to consider with regard to medication than timers and dosages. L-dopa, the drug traditionally used to treat Parkinson's, like any drug, it has its drawbacks, namely a side effect known as dyskinesia.

Dyskinesia presents as a sudden jerking movement in the limbs and typically manifests when L-dopa has built up in a person's system, usually after a 'honeymoon period' of about five years. For an older person with Parkinson's, it might make sense to approach the disease with lifestyle modifications, saving L-dopa for later in treatment to sustain a quality of life. For someone my age, waiting might feel wasteful, especially when it comes to earning potential, familial responsibilities and creating a financial cushion for retirement. In any case, the participant assumes the risk.

Where L-dopa creates sudden unintentional movements, a class of drugs known as dopamine agonists report reduced rates of early-onset motor complications, but also a one-in-six chance of developing an impulse control disorder (ICD). Problems run the gamut from gambling and overspending to hypersexuality and becoming obsessed with hobbies. These issues come on slowly and can be pretty insidious, so it's crucial to be aware of any behavioural changes and to keep the lines of communication open with your family, friends and care team.

With no panacea, it's up to me to meet this disease halfway. For now, I decide to give the dopamine agonists a wide berth. The urge to splurge is an occupational hazard in my line of work. I certainly don't fancy waking up in a cold sweat surrounded by Brown Thomas receipts, having blown €20,000 on designer gear. Although L-dopa presents similar risks, the odds don't seem as high in my inexpert opinion.

Dr Sweeney suggests some helpful tools, like keeping a daily symptoms journal for patterns particular to my Parkinson's journey. "I haven't kept a diary since I was a kid," I admit, cringing at the pages I dedicated to my secondary school crush, John Scally. If memory serves me, it had a lock and key and reeked of vanilla body spray.

Times, I will quickly learn, are important. Times I take my tablets. Times I feel my symptoms kick in. Times I get my monthly cycle. Everything is connected. There is data in the everyday. Who knows? Maybe having meticulously documented the number of times John Scally looked at me in class will serve me well in this era of my life.

As a single woman who lives alone, I spend a lot of time planning for and thinking about the future. It worries me that Parkinson's is progressive and incurable, so I ask Dr Sweeney what happens if my condition worsens to the point where my quality of life is affected? I'd like to know what my options are.

We discuss deep brain stimulation (DBS), a neurosurgical procedure involving the implantation of electrodes in the brain. Used to treat motor symptoms in people with more advanced Parkinson's and those with a poor response to other therapies, DBS has been shown to ease symptoms such as dyskinesia, tremor, rigidity and walking problems. The risks are high, but so is the payoff in improving a person's quality of life. It is now being lauded as a pre-emptive treatment for people with early-onset Parkinson's who are, like myself, tremor-dominant. Why? Tremors don't always respond as effectively to L-dopa as other motor symptoms.

Of course, something of this magnitude takes time. There is an embargo of several years from diagnosis before being permitted treatment, not to mention a lengthy waiting list. Then there are tests to determine physical and psychological eligibility, plus pre- and post-operative preparation and hospital visits. Dr Sweeney assures me that if my motor skills hypothetically worsen to the point where surgery is necessary, chances are that non-surgical options might already be available.

To me, he seems genuinely optimistic about the latest research and technological breakthroughs, from focused ultrasound stimulation to implanting a small electrode stimulator in the arm, both of which help to ease motor symptoms for up to a year. The upshot? Not having to undergo invasive procedures like DBS.

More fascinating still is a field of study where neurologists are spotting Parkinson's motor symptoms *before* they physically manifest. He tells us about a study involving a soccer player with Parkinson's where neurologists were able to spot apparently early signs pre-dating obvious physical symptoms by ten years.

Today is a very different day from when we first met. I am motivated by a new world of possibilities. I hardly know Dr Sweeney, but I already know I trust him. I also trust my intuition, which is telling me to start on L-dopa medication for all the reasons he cites and for no other reason than to prove to myself that this is, indeed, Parkinson's.

He writes me a script and schedules a follow-up phone call after Christmas to see how I'm getting on with the medication. In the meantime, he arranges for me to have a DaTscan and to see the CUH physiotherapist, who has a specific interest in Parkinson's.

Before wrapping up, we exchange season's greetings and best wishes for 2022. With phones back on, a jumble of pings and alerts remind us we are needed elsewhere. Julie gets the car warmed up while I sign out at reception. Once outside the convent doors, I remove my mask. Finally, I can breathe again. Inhaling deeper than usual, I allow a ripple of satisfaction to escape. It's been a good day. I turn the corner of the building towards Julie's car, hand rifling through my bag – the usual lucky dip routine. Then I spot it, solo and sovereign: a tulip near one of the oak trees, claiming space in a barren season.

* * *

The mood is lighter on the way home, partly because we know our route and don't have to listen to the passive-aggressive backseat driver on Google Maps, but mostly because there's a sense of relief and direction where once there was none.

Julie successfully navigates the serpentine roads as the traffic lights ahead of us turn green. "I'm so relieved for you, Annie. You have options. This is like a Christmas miracle!"

"I think the Virgin Mary has dibs on that," I wager, taking another lucky dip in my bag for God knows what, "but it's certainly miracle adjacent." I pull out a bottle of water and try opening it. "I read somewhere the other day that you don't die *from* Parkinson's, you die *with* it."

"Oh, dear. I think Parkinson's needs a new publicist," she laughs, gesturing for me to hand her the bottle. I comply, bested by rigid fingers. "How about, 'You don't die from it, you live with it?'" She loosens the cap and hands it back.

"Well, a lot depends on the delivery," I muse between sips. "Otherwise, it could be like my last Christmas FM Classical show. I was introducing the hymn, 'What Child Is This?' It sounded like someone forgot to pick baby Jesus up from crèche."

"Oh, Annie!" She shakes her head. "Remind me never to have you do the school run."

While swapping anecdotes and key points from the outpatient meeting, we both agree that I'm in expert hands with Dr Sweeney. His ability to retain facts is especially impressive; you can immediately sense his passion and purpose in doing what he does.

I share nuggets of online research I discovered over the weekend thanks to Parkinson's Ireland, a national non-profit support group for people with Parkinson's.

"They've got some useful information about how women experience the disease. I didn't realise we get a double whammy of low dopamine every month due to hormonal fluctuations. So, every time I ovulate or menstruate, I might also face a spike in symptoms. And I'll probably have forgotten this by the time I get home, courtesy of this damned brain fog."

"Perimenopause!" we shout in unison as I clench my fists like Maria Callas in a rendition of "Vedi, ecco, vedi". I told you we were drama queens.

"You know, it might be useful to connect with other people with Parkinson's, especially women experiencing the same thing," Julie says. "Do you know of any meetups or support groups in Cork?"

"Not off the top of my head," I admit. "Although, I don't expect I will. Not now, anyway. The past few days have been intense, but today was a real turning point. It felt like lockdown lifting all over again: that sense of my old life returning, or the closest thing possible. To be truthful, Jules, I just want to take my medication and get on with it."

"Of course. I can only imagine. It could be worth looking into when you're ready." She shoots me an understanding smile.

One foot in front of the other.

* * *

The next few days are magic. I collect my medication, meet friends and family and bask in the glow of possibilities, guided by my North Star – naivety.

You'll soon understand what I mean. Not everything lasts. Even joy is fleeting. Why else would we grieve its passing? While we're here, let's just enjoy the moment. We never know what's next.

To think I spent almost a year and a half afraid of catching COVID, not knowing I had Parkinson's. I feared COVID's impact on my career as work ground to a halt, unaware of what was to have the final blow. The spontaneity that defined pre-pandemic life would eventually return, only to be snatched from my grasp in ways I never imagined. COVID put my life on pause, but Parkinson's razed it to rubble, smiled and said, "Start again".

CHAPTER THREE

Drugs

One size does not fit all

January 2022

I'M LYING IN BED, arms by my side, wearing a thick white duvet like a strapless gown. A veil of light diffuses through the curtains, giving the darkness a ceremonial glow. Tonight, I'm going to sleep just like last night and the night before. Of that, I am certain. Two weeks ago, things were much different, but since starting medication, my symptoms are negligible, besides the odd flutter in my hand. It's working. I know like I know. And I know I have Parkinson's.

Drifting into a semi-slumber, I sense something in my left shoulder. A twitch followed by a slight jerk. Again. Then nothing. Then again. My limbs tighten and my eyes open. I switch on the bedside lamp and grab my phone, forgetting the commitment to my pillow.

Swipe. Search.

"What is dyskinesia?" *Involuntary sporadic movements.*

That's what I thought, but this may not happen for at least another five years. "Why the left side?" I worry. "Why now?" Keen to get back to sleep, I make a mental note to email

Dr Sweeney and try dozing off, but the moment has passed. Instead, I pull off my strapless gown, shuffle into the kitchen and make a cup of tea.

*   *   *

I have time on my hands, it being January and all. Workwise, I write my usual Saturday column for the *Irish Examiner*, but not much else. Kids are still off school and most folks remain in post-Christmas hibernation. The modest workflow is a welcome reprieve from the intensity of December, a chance to exhale and get familiar with the day-to-day details of life with Parkinson's.

I'm marking up my bullet journal – a gift to myself – Monday through Sunday, with time bands correlating to my daily medication doses and exercise goals. Beneath each band is a note section for anything specific to that day, such as whether I'm sick or have my monthly cycle – the anecdotal information that complements black-and-white facts.

I recall Dr Sweeney discussing the importance of taking L-dopa on time and something called 'wearing off' periods, when the average four-to-five-hour window of relief from symptoms gets smaller. If adjustments need to be made to my dosage and medication times, having this hard data to hand makes life a lot simpler. On Andy's advice, I've started using a medication alarm app that also logs each dose down to the minute. Combined with my new Fitbit, which records sleep, hydration, calories and hourly activity, I'm in danger of becoming a human flowchart.

Talk is cheap, so I lace up my trainers, grab my parka and get a start on those 10,000 steps. Today's bright and breezy weather is tailor-made for a brisk 'walk' up the hellscape in

Cork known as Coach Hill. Self-loathing is the only vehicle (aside from a four-wheel drive) that will propel you to the top, but the panoramic view of Douglas estuary transitioning from land to sea is worth the side stitches and joint strain.

The loop usually takes me the guts of an hour at a slightly breathless pace. Having left the apartment at 11.45 a.m., I reach the tail end of Maryborough Hill, just across from Julie's house, around 12.30 p.m. As I turn the corner to face the fifteen-minute home stretch, I feel shaky. My alarm goes off, alerting me to the second yellow pill of the day, which I realise I forgot to bring with me. *No worries*, I say to myself. *A quarter of an hour shouldn't hurt.*

By the time I exit the elevator to my apartment, I am trembling uncontrollably.

I make four vain attempts to put my key in the door before divine intervention does the honours. My jelly legs find their way to the medicine cabinet, where I fumble with the child-proof bottle for several awkward seconds before swallowing my yellow tablet with a gulp of water. It takes another 20 to 30 minutes before the dopamine kicks in, during which time I sit on the toilet seat, happy to rest against the cold cistern and wait for stillness to descend.

A few days later, Andy sends me a metal pill container for my keychain – a freebie he got from the chemist. I fill the cylinder to the top and attach it to the bundle of fobs and keys hanging on a hook beside the front door. This, my friends, is known as a 'teachable moment'.

* * *

My Auntie Margaret (Mom's sister and, yes, another Margaret) puts me in touch with her friend, Marie – the chairperson of a local Parkinson's chapter. "She can help," she tells me. That she does.

When I call her, she lets me talk for 45 minutes while I do that thing I do – overshare. It's a pandemic habit I can't seem to shake, perpetuated by too much time spent alone. Now, I'm *that* person. The one who talks to cab drivers, chats with the UPS delivery guys, chews the fat at the supermarket check-out – *even when it's self-service*. Bear with me. I'm working on it.

With over 20 years' experience assisting the Parkinson's community, her advice is incredibly practical. First and foremost, I must get my medication right. This takes time and will require regular adjustments, but it's worth the effort from the start. Next are things like nutrition, hydration, sleep and exercise. Like it or not, healthful lifestyle modifications support treatment efficacy and help alleviate symptoms. I consider myself in fairly good nick but, given half a chance, I could live on caffeine and sugar. Finally, once I get my body and mind used to this new way of living, only then should I consider attending a support group. Every individual case of Parkinson's is different. At this early point in my journey, seeing someone whose condition depreciates could set me back a few steps.

I take her point. By nature, I process things on my own anyway. I'm sure I'll figure it out. That said, if I get wind of the fact that they serve pastries at Parkinson's coffee mornings, I won't be held responsible for the actions of my sweet tooth. In the meantime, Marie takes my address so that she can send me some literature on eating and living well with Parkinson's.

A few days later, two booklets arrive in my letterbox with nutritional tips and information about Parkinson's-adjacent matters such as bone health, difficulty swallowing and unintentional weight loss. Photos of seniors living their best lives smile back at me from every second page. Despite my recent diagnosis, I unconsciously internalise the advice as something that affects other people, not me. In my head, being healthy and having Parkinson's are mutually exclusive, with three yellow tablets in between – for the time being, at least.

* * *

Andy and Neil collect me from my first physio appointment at CUH, where I undergo a battery of tests to assess my gait, balance and coordination. Considering the past issues with my right side, there is nothing of immediate concern. I'm thrilled, even more so because the boys will be staying for the weekend. When we arrive at the apartment car park, Andy grabs their overnight bags from the back seat of the SUV while Neil ferrets around in the boot and extracts a large, branded bag from Nolan's delicatessen in Clontarf. Some things never change.

Inside the kitchen, Neil lays out the magical delicacies: burrata cheese; the charcuterie staples of prosciutto, pancetta, chorizo, olives and antipasti; fresh sourdough bread and balsamic vinegar; artisan nuts dipped in salted caramel. Oh, and wine – lots of wine. Andy grabs a bottle of Pinot Noir. "See, we were thinking of you," he nods, showcasing the screw cap and pours three glasses for a long overdue "Cheers".

"I went to Aldi this morning," Andy tells us while Neil meticulously studies what's missing from the posh buffet, "and some aul lad was staring at the jams for five minutes. I think he was looking for the third secret of Fatima."

"Excuse me. I'm right beside you!" Neil fake reprimands Andy, whose naughty laugh fills the room. It's like old times.

"This is snack food, by the way," Neil mentions. "Dinner is booked for 6 p.m. at Da Mirco on Bridge Street – a bit earlier so it doesn't interfere with your evening dose." Boys after my own heart.

Andy assumes a comfy seat in the Eames chair, takes another sip of his drink and does what he does best: assess.

"What are your utility bills like, Ams? You know you can change service providers after a year? Give me a look at your unit price and I can sort that out for you."

You always know where you stand with Andy. He is easy to read and reads people easily. With a Stanley blade on the edge of his tongue, cross him and he'll cut you with his words before breakfast. He's also a loyal friend who never wants you to pay above asking, who'll rent a van in the middle of a storm to help you move, who'll let you stash your worldly belongings in his spare room for the guts of a year and who, behind the incessant questioning similar to my sisters', is motivated purely by love.

"I was going to ask you in the car, but I thought I'd wait until you had a drink in front of you," he says in his classic acerbic tone. "How is the new medication going?"

"Good, overall," I reply. "I've only been taking the tablets for three weeks, so I'm still getting used to it."

"Any side effects?" Neil asks as we each claim a section of the sofa.

"A bit," I reply.

"Like a bit pregnant? Come on, Ams." Andy's disapproving stare says it all.

"I've been getting spontaneous involuntary movements from the L-dopa, which is common but not typical for someone recently diagnosed."

"Have you spoken to your consultant?"

Andy can see it in my guilty expression. "Not yet."

Neil puts a bowl of macadamia nuts on the table. "Look, I know you've been through the wringer," he sympathises, "but you've got to keep asking those questions. Your diagnosis is only the start of things." Andy nods in agreement.

I slump deeper into the upholstery. "It's been 16 months of guessing. I thought I'd have a chance to catch my breath and live my life again for a little while, at least."

"It doesn't work that way," Andy remarks, delivering the final piece of tough love. "I don't know much about Parkinson's, but I'm pretty sure when it comes to anything progressive, you better get used to finding your voice."

Andy is right. I don't reach out enough. I don't speak up for myself. I put up and shut up, not wanting to be a burden. There may be no right way of doing Parkinson's, but it can't hurt to be more vocal.

* * *

The following afternoon, we drive to Monkstown and walk along the waterfront, looking out at Cobh. From afar, the sailboats look like toothpicks bobbing in the harbour. The breeze feels good. Pity I can't say the same for me – the dizziness, the nausea. It's awful. Plus, all I did was toss and turn last night. I should know better. Alcohol before bed isn't the smartest idea, especially when it's combined with medication that could amplify the symptoms of a hangover or restless legs.

We cross the road to The Bosun pub to meet our friends Olly and Alan – fellow Dublin immigrants who, like me, recently crossed the Jack Lynch Tunnel and never looked back. Orders of fish, chips, mushy peas and pints fill our table. I opt for water, barely picking at the food on my plate.

"You OK, Ams?" whispers Neil while the others are mid-conversation.

I shake my head, afraid to open my mouth.

"You look pale. Try and eat something."

My eyes say "sorry". This was supposed to be a fun weekend of making memories, not me mainlining aspirin.

I keep forgetting that nothing phases Neil. Considering we met in 1998 after my then-flatmate introduced us, he has a lot of material – nay, archives – should he ever wish to blackmail me. Not that he ever would.

Neil is the kind of guy who sends chocolates and champagne to your office the day before your birthday. The kind of guy who patiently reads every terrible draft of your novel and who listens to your ten-minute voice notes without deleting them unread. He can hold court on any subject, from world politics to trashy internet gossip, all the while making space for you to share what's on your mind and heart. When he speaks his truth, it is never at the expense of someone's feelings. He is one of the few people who has ever seen my soft underbelly. He is the person I trust. Everyone should have a Neil.

"Hey, we'll be leaving shortly," he reassures me. "If you need to go to bed early when we get home, go ahead. Forget about us. It's just Andy and me. This isn't *The Real Housewives*."

"But you're my guests," I sigh.

"Ams, we came to support you, not be waited on. You aren't being judged on your hosting skills. And more to the point, no one will flip a table should you miss the mark."

"Well, maybe Andy."

A shared smirk belies the meaningful moment. We glance across the table to see him in his signature puffer and denim shorts regaling Olly and Alan. Someone's ears are ringing, for sure.

"Look, you're bound to have a few more of these 'off' days, whatever they may look like, but their lived experience will also be etched in your brain. There's so much to take in;

everything you do now needs to be double-checked and signed off by you: when to sleep, what to eat, what *not* to eat . . ." We both look at the plates of deep-fried food in front of us, mine virtually untouched. "See," he gestures in my direction without missing a beat, "you're doing great already.

"My point is, go easy on yourself. Your whole lifestyle is changing. You're allowed to make mistakes. It's part of the learning curve. You know you always have us. We're your biggest cheerleaders, but we can't do this for you. You've got to make yourself your main priority."

That evening, I go to bed early.

* * *

February 2022

When Neil and Andy leave the following day, I get cosy on the sofa and watch the movie *Love & Other Drugs* on Netflix. Why I decide to watch this *alone* is anyone's guess. The protagonist, Maggie Murdock (played by Anne Hathaway), is a free-spirited server with early-onset Parkinson's. Her love interest, Jamie Randall (played by Jake Gyllenhaal), is a slick pharma sales rep with chronic playboy-itis. During their first date scene, I can't help but notice Maggie's tremor. Correction: I *can't* notice Maggie's tremor. A delicate quiver, like that of a fledgling ballerina, its presence is almost poetic, despite Jamie's cheesy one-liners, which are enough to cause anyone to twitch. Speaking of which, might they have picked a better job for our protagonist? Last I checked, hot coffee and uncontrollable body movements do not a copacetic pairing make.

But what do I know? Close to 50 and terminally single, my partner-picking skills are in worse shape than my dopamine levels. Lightning doesn't strike twice, so since I've already ticked the rare disease box, my chance of meeting someone special is looking delusional. Even if I do fall in love, there's the clear and present reality of an incurable brain disorder, and three is a crowd. In sickness and in health, but what if the prospect is too much? What if *I'm* not enough? What then?

Then comes the part in the movie where Jamie attends a neurology conference and meets a man whose wife has late-stage Parkinson's. Upon discovering that Jamie's girlfriend, Maggie, is only in the early stages of the disease, he offers him some sobering advice:

> Go upstairs, pack your bags and leave a nice note. Find yourself a healthy woman. I love my wife. I do. But I wouldn't do it over again. The thing nobody tells you, this disease will steal everything you love in her. Her body, her smile, her mind. Sooner or later, she'll lose motor control. Eventually, she won't even be able to dress herself. Then, the fun really begins. Cleaning up her shit. Frozen face. Dementia. It's not a disease, it's a Russian novel.

He's right, you know. I've been living with Parkinson's for 16 months – my longest committed relationship. Being told I have an incurable neurodegenerative disease isn't exactly the meet-cute I imagined. As for sharing a life? It's challenging, to say the least: the uncontrollable movements, the pain, the sleepless nights, needing medication just to get by. And the compromises are all on my end.

Like Maggie, I don't want to need someone. I especially don't want to need someone to care for me. I might look independent on the outside, but I'm a loner on the inside –

an amateur at fostering long-term commitments and a pro at getting spooked. Psychology calls this style of relating 'avoidant attachment'. TikTok calls it a 'red flag'. I call it 'self-preservation'. But at what price? Being alone for the rest of my life? With my health privileges revoked, I can't afford to be independent. If I want a happily ever after, I have to learn to let people in.

Even if I invite someone to share my day-to-day, I don't see them staying. Life is no longer romantic or spontaneous. It is prosaic, tedious and it takes a metric tonne of stamina simply to 'manage' my condition – something which Parkinson's depletes at will. Each day rolls out with military-like precision, from meals to medication, sleep, exercise and hydration. Even leaving the house requires tactical mapping and a time-bound plan.

There are no dinner reservations at eight if my next dose is at nine. No second date if I can't walk a straight line or order a round of drinks without trembling. No casual sleepovers without having extra medication to hand. No deep and meaningful chats if I'm suddenly 'off-peak' or in the throes of excessive daytime sleepiness. The fact is, I now come first, which makes little room for catering to someone else's needs. How can I share a future with someone when my own is measured out in milligrams?

I watch the movie's closing scene of the couple as they live and love together in their wood-beamed loft apartment, signalling joy and hope. Still, I can't help interpreting Jamie's final soliloquy with a deep absence in my heart: "Sometimes, the thing you want most doesn't happen. And sometimes, the thing you never expect does."

Parkinson's and I: We're in it for the long haul. 'Til death do us part.

March 2022

Six weeks have passed since my come-to-Jesus moment with Neil and Andy. Things seem to be OK so far, bar the dyskinesia in my left shoulder and gradual reprisal of nocturnal movements. To be fair, I don't mind the occasional body popping – it's a conversation starter – but the midnight dance parties I could do without. And so, my prescription now includes a pink slow-release pill to continue the stream of dopamine in my system and smooth out the edges while I sleep. This gives me the confidence to attend a press trip to Madeira with the Portuguese Tourist Board. The change of scenery will do me good. Plus, it's my second time there. The familiarity will balance out the newness of managing my symptoms and medication on a packed itinerary around people I don't know. It's also an opportunity to gauge their reactions when I tell them I have Parkinson's – a 'soft launch', as it were.

On arrival at Dublin Airport, I'm already exhausted. Reports of 90-minute security clearance times see travellers arriving three-and-a-half hours in advance to catch their flights – which in my case is on the back of a four-hour Aircoach journey from Cork.

A smooth landing on Funchal's notoriously inhospitable runway makes up for the late take-off. After a lovely welcome dinner at a local restaurant, I get situated in my hotel room and go to bed. Two hours later, I wake with restless legs, bilateral jerking and foot spasms so bad that I have no choice but to get up and pace the room. I try a few downward dog yoga poses to no avail, besides rug burn on my matless hands. Then I take two ibuprofen tablets with some herbal tea, but they have no discernible effect. Fed up, I get back into bed and assume the foetal position as if these aggressive movements will lull me back to sleep.

Up before sunrise, I soothe myself with a hot shower before applying fake lashes to awaken my eyes, which, at this point, resemble cigarette burns. I do some research on today's schedule; thankfully it involves food, wine tasting and a relaxing stroll in the Monte Palace tropical garden. At a loose end, I walk down to the hotel dining room a bit too early, planning to sit in the common area until breakfast is served at 6 a.m. I like to be among the few pioneers claiming the first exotic fruits and freshly baked bread before the gaggle of prospectors descends later.

There's a strange phenomenon on press trips. Like arriving in a foreign country on a college exchange programme, you bond instantly with a group of strangers for a short period and, in most cases, never see them again. My recent habit of over-disclosure serves me well in this scenario, as a fellow journalist joins me for breakfast and asks me how I slept. He offers me some Solpadeine, which his wife packed for him, knowing he'd have a few pints, and I gratefully accept them. The codeine should help me nod off tonight or fall back to sleep if need be. Good or bad, I don't care. I want to enjoy the views of the scenic waterfalls and breathtaking aqueduct walks, not be nodding off in the back of a jeep or feeling too wiped to hold a conversation. Besides, it's my job to write about my experience, which I can't do if it is shrouded in low-level anxiety about insomnia.

After dinner each evening, the gang goes out for drinks; some go dancing and others go to the casino. I don't join them. On our last night, I prefer to return to the hotel where I can check in online for tomorrow's flight home and bank some valuable shuteye. *Is this me?* I ask myself. *Early nights, earlier mornings, not joining in on the fun?* Then, I think back to what Neil said, "Put yourself first," and Andy's advice about being more vocal. Although giving my medication tweaks some time to bed-in before concluding if they work or not is standard, I should probably share this information. I'm blessed with a communicative and caring consultant whom I can ring or email without having to attend the outpatient department for changes to be made. Maybe it's an Irish thing, but I always feel like I'm putting people out, even when they make it clear that I'm not. I put a reminder in my calendar to connect with Dr Sweeney when I get home, double-check I've ticked priority boarding and press 'confirm'.

April 2022

Some lessons need to be learned the hard way. I arrive back in Cork for a day's turnaround before heading to Dublin to style a photoshoot. I could use the money, and I am happy to be back even though the timing is tight. A day's prep followed by a day's shooting is not uncommon, but it demands all of you for those 48 hours. And the weather. Oh, the weather. It's as if Mother Nature has a vendetta. Incessant gales and rain elevate stress levels as she threatens to damage bags of clothes en route from retailers. Like a sniper, she waits until the camera is ready to click before a bitter gust runs ramshackle through the model's hair, making her eyes water and legs turn blueish pink. The intense schedule and inclement conditions, combined with the usual few hours that pass for sleep, all but deplete my battery. Awash with adrenaline, I don't feel the energy whiplash until I am back home, where I spend the better part of a week splayed out on my sofa. Neil's words about putting my needs first ring in my ear. When it comes to energy management – a common Parkinson's complaint – it's clear I'm not doing anything to help mine, but I need to work. I need the cash flow. I need to feel like the 'old me'.

Weeks of broken sleep follow. I wake every night with restless legs and feet – painful and burning with pins and needles. The discomfort leaves me no choice but to get out of bed and walk around to ease the 'wearing off' sensation, when dopamine is at its lowest. The pink pill that usually does a full night's shift clocks off early, now giving me three to five hours' grace – if I'm lucky. Those painful, restless legs follow me during the day as I sit at my desk trying to work and the articles I need to file remain firmly on the long, shaky finger. Concentration is an art form. To top it all, the dyskinesia in my shoulder now affects my neck and head. I am in a constant state of movement, so I nap intermittently to keep myself recharged. Otherwise, I'm fit for nothing. This irks me. I'm not the type of person to do nothing. Nothing is a zero-sum game, and I'm not very good at losing. I didn't build a life I love over the past 49 years to have Parkinson's carelessly take it away. Right now, I don't need to accept another work project. I need to get my medication adjusted. I need to avoid burning out. Most of all, I need to redefine 'need'.

May 2022

We are mid-chinwag, Julie and I, our mugs of tea now cold from neglect. There is so much to catch up on, with her daughter Lara's confirmation this Saturday and our college friends coming to Cork. I try reaching the switch on the kettle from my breakfast bar perch. Julie interrupts.

"Annie, how are you feeling?"

"I've been better," I reply, double-crossed by stiffness and twitching. "I'm waking during the night with hot, painful, restless legs *and* feet on both sides of my body. It's happening during the day, too." The kettle wins, forcing me off my stool and into the kitchen.

"The dose of L-dopa that used to get me through the night now only lasts about five hours. It's exhausting. I find I have a finite amount of energy during the day, after which I'm completely drained unless I have a nap," I explain. The water comes to a boil.

"And that's not the half of it. The jerking in my arm now affects my neck, shoulder and head at times. I was on a video call with Maureen last Sunday and she noticed it. I looked like one of those bobbling toy dogs you stick on a car dashboard. Poor Mo," I sigh. "Her calls always turn into ad hoc therapy sessions. There's always some new level of fuckery with this bloody condition. I used to walk the seafront path from Rochestown to Monkstown and back, no bother. Now, I can't go to the corner shop without feeling spent."

Julie's straight face starts to slip as I pour the kettle.

"It's also a *total* pain in the arse trying to figure out what are Parkinson's symptoms or medication side effects. Only recently, I started on an additional drug; it's an anti-depressant with sleep-promoting effects," I explain, "but I felt worse, so I stopped taking it."

"Jesus, Annie. You can't live or work like that."

"I know. That's why I'm giving up styling. I simply can't do it anymore. I'm a liability. Safety pins, zips, ribbons, clasps, buttons – it's like an assault course for my fine-motor skills, only the poor model is the one getting the bashing. The whole world now has Zoom fatigue, so my online services are dead in the water. As for writing jobs, I'm afraid to take on anything new in case I miss a deadline. Vickie, my boss in the *Examiner*, has been so accommodating and understanding, but we have a 14-year relationship. She knows me. I don't have that bond with a new client."

I hand Julie her green tea as I try to locate the missing box of Barry's.

"How are you managing to pay for your apartment?"

My stomach lurches. "Savings," I reveal. "I have a small emergency fund, but most emergencies happen in an instant and they're done – like an accident, an unexpected surgery or a bill. This feels indefinite." Both of us know this doesn't end well.

"I sound bone practical," Julie owns up, as if priming me for something out of character, "but have you considered a more secure job? Maybe an administrative role in the public sector? Something with guaranteed pay that isn't too taxing?"

I deposit one of the missing teabags into my mug. "Don't you remember that office temping job back in the day where I mistakenly gave pension payments to their construction workers? I was demoted to the filing cabinet by early morning and relieved of my duties by noon. And that was long before Parkinson's."

"Annie, I'm serious. You have no guarantees right now – not your health, your job, your living situation – and it's frightening, to be quite honest."

"I understand your point, Jules," I agree, "but I don't think I would be an ideal candidate for a nine-to-five role. Dr Sweeney and I already discussed possible remedies like DBS surgery at my last outpatient appointment, with my tremor being in the small percentage that doesn't fully respond to L-dopa. It was only worst-case scenario but still.

"Do you know I spent two days a week this month alone attending health-related appointments? That's not factoring in how much longer it takes me to complete a task when my motor symptoms are active or when I haven't slept, which is every damn day."

"This must be so infuriating for you," she sighs. "It's like you're going around in circles. I'm so glad you live in a rent-pressure zone. I get a knot in my stomach when I hear stories about landlords hiking up rents with barely any notice or ending a lease so they can increase the monthly ask. It's disgraceful."

"You needn't worry. Patricia is already making mental plans to convert the garage into a granny flat. Should I want it or need it in the future, it's there."

"Well, that's a relief. At least you'll always have somewhere to live. You don't look so thrilled, though."

I smile with mild disappointment. "Have you ever felt flattered and flattened all at once?"

No answer.

"What I mean is . . . I mean . . . I'm immensely grateful. I just never imagined my life as a decrepit spinster living in my sister's garage. That's not exactly what I had on my vision board. I feel ashamed I couldn't make it on my own. Miss So-Called Independent: a total farce. Laughable, even.

"I keep thinking, where did I go wrong? What if I chose a more solid career path or got married and had kids? How would my life have turned out? Would this moment even exist, or would I be somewhere like Zermatt in Switzerland, getting red-light therapy at a wellness lodge to optimise my treatment? Look, it's not like my old life was comparable to Anna Wintour's, but it was mine. I created it. And now it's slipping through my fingers."

Julie reaches for words that aren't there.

"You don't have to say anything," I insist. "The truth is you are right. I don't have the luxury of choice anymore. Who knows how quickly before becomes after? One minute I'm drinking tea with you and making plans for Saturday, and the next I'm in physio twice a week due to a fall or with an occupational therapist because I've lost my ability to speak."

"That will never happen, Annie – the speaking bit, that is."

Peals of laughter ease the tension. "I'm my mother's daughter. Of that, there's no doubt. Everything else is up for grabs."

"Out of interest," Julie asks, softening her register. "What would you have done differently?"

"Before or after my diagnosis?"

"Before."

"I wouldn't have been so afraid."

* * *

At my next outpatient appointment with Dr Sweeney, I tell him about my symptoms and ask if it is a progression of the disease. He reassures me that it's a matter of getting the balance right with medication, particularly for a busy, active person. A few tweaks are made to the dosage and frequency to help sustain the dopamine in my body. We discuss adjunctive support in more detail, like dopamine agonists, which are particularly well-suited to newly diagnosed tremor-dominant patients like me, who have no cognitive impairment, but also useful in advanced patients with a tremor that is resistant to L-dopa. Another class of medication called anticholinergics can also reduce symptoms by blocking a brain chemical that influences movement. It's not a name I easily remember, but one I soon won't forget. Although dopamine agonists sound promising, I can't say the same about their worrisome caveat: a 1 in 6 chance of acquiring an impulse control disorder (ICD). Compared to winning the lottery (1 in 10.7 million), getting pregnant after 40 (1 in 20) or dying in a car accident (1 in 84), the odds of developing an ICD are quite good. I'm not a betting gal, but my intuition tells me now's probably not the best time to start. So, I put this on hold until we assess all other options.

While on the subject of successful but scary remedies, we revisit deep brain stimulation (DBS) surgery and its pre-emptive use for those (especially early-onset) who might have a smaller window of relief from 'on-off' movement fluctuations. As I've only been experiencing symptoms for one-and-a-half years, I don't meet the current criteria for potential candidates, but given the waiting list size, it might be worth submitting my name for consideration. Should my motor symptoms persist, I'll at least be in the queue. Worst case scenario, of course. I table this along with dopamine agonists for the time being, happy to have my medication sorted and my DaTscan completed the previous day. One foot in front of the other.

* * *

I collect my new prescription from the chemist along with a large pill organiser and some laxatives before making my way to the adjacent bus stop. Constipation, would you believe, is one of the first pre-clinical signs of Parkinson's disease and one of the most frequent non-motor symptoms in people with Parkinson's. It's also a side effect of the medication. Dopamine controls toilet habits: who knew? A lot of folks don't because, well, who wants to talk about bowel movements?

To keep things in working order, I take one that's non-dependency forming when needed, which is almost daily and with no guarantee of success. I can handle that. What I find hard to deal with is the laxative itself – a cloying syrup which, even though having a sweet tooth, is hard to stomach. Speaking of which, the bloating isn't exactly a joy ride either.

Case in point: today. I look like I'm seven months pregnant. Everything I wear feels tight, aside from leggings and my oversized roll-neck sweater. Even my socks hurt. Most annoyingly, a sugary film covers my front teeth – a souvenir from my last capful which only a thorough brushing seems to shift. Lovely.

Joining the waiting commuters, I check my travel app to discover the 220 to Carrigaline will be another 12 minutes. In mid-afternoon traffic, that's a solid 20, so to pass the time, I retrieve my new gadget from my leather tote bag. The word 'gadget' might be overselling it. The pill organiser is more like something you find in nursing homes: a plastic case filled with moulded containers marked Monday to Sunday and sections for morning, mid-morning, afternoon and evening doses. It feels so . . . clinical.

It's not that deep, I tell myself. *Just pretend it's for vitamins.*

My eyes immediately start to well up. I'm not great at pretending. Embarrassed, I turn my back to the half dozen people looking down at their phones and use my sleeve to absorb the tears. Rummaging in my pockets for a tissue, the sound of Mozart's Piano Sonata No. 12 wafts softly from my bag. It's Margaret.

"Hey, sweetheart. How are you?"

"Hi," I croak.

"What's wrong? Talk to me." I move around the corner for privacy and prop my head against the stone wall, its uneven surface kneading the knots of tension.

"You just caught me at a bad time, that's all," I say, still holding onto my silicone-covered future.

"I bought myself a pill organiser so that I'm on top of my meds . . . and laxatives which are now par for the course."

Margaret knows to wait a beat.

"Mags, I feel so . . . old!" I sob. "How did I get here? I'm only in my forties. I don't know how to navigate this."

She issues another big-sister-approved "Oh, sweetheart" and lets me let it all out.

"Honestly, I'm not looking for sympathy. I just feel a bit overwhelmed. This is my life now – pills and not being able to poop!" An elderly gentleman passes in earshot of my complaint and gives a sympathetic head tilt. He knows the drill.

"I try telling myself they are no different to vitamins—"

"But they're not," she interjects. "They keep your brain and body functioning. This is real. You're allowed to feel jarred."

"In the privacy of my apartment, Mags." I check my app to see if the bus is near, too mortified to peer around the corner after my emotional display.

"If it makes you feel better, years ago, my HHT flared up while I was in the ladies' room at a restaurant on a date. I had the mother of all nosebleeds. Nothing would stop it. I was in there for about half an hour. The guy thought I ghosted him."

"What did you do?"

"I had to pack the inside of my nose with tissue and walk out of the toilets looking like I had gone ten rounds with an MMA fighter."

"Did you explain?"

"I had no other choice. Imagine what was going through his head! We wound up dating after that."

Tears turn quickly to laughter, so much so that I almost miss my bus. Humour, for the record, is a proven tonic and is available without a prescription. I highly recommend it.

June 2022

When it comes to sleep, eight and a half hours is my sweet spot. Anything less than seven hours and I'm barely able to spell my name or tell you where I live. Not only am I a long sleeper, I'm also a deep sleeper. I'll sleep through parties, arguments, home renovations – you name it. As for naps, I take them daily and maintain they should be a constitutional right.

This was before Parkinson's hit, though. Now it's more like this: three to five hours is my sweet spot. Anything more than six hours and I am campaigning to call it a public holiday. Not only am I a light sleeper, I'm also a fitful one, waking up when my body throws shapes during the night, deciding it wants to let loose. As for naps, I take them daily. I have no choice. Sunken eyes and dark circles aren't a good look for me.

The reason I'm so tired? Parkinson's likes to party. It likes insomnia. It likes to mess with your REM cycle. Then, it likes you to re-enact your dreams. Failing that, some juicy nightmares will do. Most of all, it likes EDS (excessive daytime sleepiness), thanks to the lived experience of the disease or the dopaminergic medications used to treat it.

Daytime, really? Oh, the bitter irony.

Over the next few weeks, I spend money I don't have on seemingly therapeutic paraphernalia I don't need: a weighted blanket, foot massager, bogus Chinese herbs from that sketchy pop-up and bee pollen, which I take out of sheer desperation when a so-called kinesiologist tells me I need more yellow in my life.

My efforts to meet my medication halfway with lifestyle aids are a total misfire, but when you can't sleep, soaking in a tonne of Epsom salts (which does nothing for my restless legs) seems reasonable. I'm curious about acupuncture, but my fear of needles gets in the way of ever giving it a go. According to research, however, it might help with relaxation and the relief of Parkinson's symptoms such as insomnia, tremors, anxiety and constipation. I figure if I could get through the past 22 months of living with Parkinson's, I can handle 30 or 40 stainless steel pins in my body and face. Right? I book my first session with a local practitioner for the following week, which feels like a sensible next step. No more throwing things at the proverbial wall, hoping they'll stick. My future decisions must be more measured than this.

In the meantime, I receive my DaTscan results, which are consistent with the clinical diagnosis of Parkinson's disease. The modicum of doubt that lingers in my brain recedes. I know like I know. According to part of the assessment, the putamen, a structure in my brain responsible for facilitating movement, is disrupted by an abnormal uptake of dopamine, which, according to my research, may also cause restless legs. I feel strangely validated when I discover this.

Ping. It's Neil.

Hey, Ams. I'm off to NYC tomorrow.

Oh, wow! You must be excited. I'm mildly jealous – won't lie!

Will get u some melatonin. How's the sleep atm?

Saw my doc. Got meds tweaked. We discussed dopamine agonists, but I took a pass. It can activate compulsions in the reward centre of the brain like deviant sexual behaviour. For now, I'm going to get some acupuncture and watch my iron levels.

Acupuncture sounds great. Can't believe you didn't opt for the deviant sexual behaviour. At the very least, you could have blamed it on the meds!

Too risky. Andy says I'll be down at the shopping centre looking for the ride. Imagine! I'd never be able to show my face in Tesco again.

Or any other bits, to be fair.

You're awful! Talk to you when you get back.

Neil doesn't know yet, but I'm taking Julie's advice and applying for a part-time copyediting job with a small consultancy to help pay the bills. I need something reliable and low stress that I can do from home and doesn't activate my symptoms. It may not be a permanent role, but after two years of a global pandemic, I'm pretty sure job security is a redundant term. In the meantime, I'm updating my LinkedIn page and removing the wardrobe and styling services from my website. Those days are over. No more chasing my old life. I've decided it's time to let it go. This is what redefining 'need' looks like.

July 2022

I'm done. Done on both sides, like a piece of burnt toast. I don't think I have the wherewithal to keep dealing with the constant demands of this condition. Some days, I feel like the personal assistant to my PD (Parkinson's Diva). Just when I think I have it under control, it throws another temper tantrum. Awkward and intransigent, it's in a constant state of defiance, waking me up in the middle of the night, insisting on separating certain foods and being a literal pain in the neck. Only this time, it's not my neck. It's a strange limp in my right leg – a mixture of heaviness and weakness when I walk. I either can't feel my thigh or it feels tremulous, along with my right calf, foot and toes which also curl inwards. When I try to wiggle them, they don't budge. The familiar pains in my feet and legs are migrating to my hands, arms and fingers. I am putting that blank space in my daily bullet journal to good use; the mainstay of symptoms appear around ovulation and before or during my monthly cycle. Stress also makes it worse.

According to my online research, musculoskeletal rigidity and reduced movement in the joints are said to be the most common source of Parkinson's pain, with severe leg pain a common complaint. Tremor has always been my primary symptom, but now the tables seem to be turning. I can't help but worry.

As my consultant is on annual leave, I'm at a loss as to who to contact. CUH doesn't have a Parkinson's nurse, and from what I know, there are only six in the country. Andy calls me later that day to catch up and asks if I've been in touch with the nurse at Parkinson's Ireland. *Of course! Why didn't I think of that?* The most obvious answer escapes my attention, which, to be fair, is rather fractured of late.

I dial the nurse hotline at Parkinson's Ireland, leaving my name and number at the beep. Lisa returns my call the following morning. She listens to me as I recount my story, from the origin of my diagnosis to my current medication plan and see-sawing symptoms. Like Dr Sweeney, she is logical yet empathetic, and she drops some home truths about what causes symptoms to worsen that I never knew about: poor sleep, when medication kicks in (peak dose) or wears off (before a tablet is due). Too much and too little medication are equally problematic, and, as I suspected, things worsen around one's monthly cycle and ovulation. Not to mention brain fog. Then, I recall the conversation I had with Julie in the car on the way back from my first outpatient appointment. Women experience the disease differently. How come I didn't make the connection? The evidence was literally written in my bullet journal – in black and white. *But the brain fog . . .*

Oh, and I've been taking my meds incorrectly – with coffee and my breakfast in the morning or on the fly and dry with what little saliva is in my mouth. Like an Olympic bobsleigh team, L-dopa needs a clear run to traverse the tricky gut–brain axis; it doesn't need a plate of scrambled eggs getting in the way. Medication should be taken a half hour before a meal or 60 to 90 minutes afterwards. As for hydration? A full glass of water is required for it to be absorbed in the gut, not to mention H_2O also helps with cognition and alleviates brain fog. If coffee and tea were water, I'd be a camel's hump. It looks like I've got some work to do.

"God, I feel silly," I cringe. "Relieved but silly."

"Why would you feel that way?" Lisa asks. "If you have a headache, do you read the leaflet that comes with the box of aspirin?"

"Er . . . no?" I half answer.

"Exactly. Not many people do. Go easy on yourself. Now you know, so take it from there."

Lisa reminds me that this diagnosis is still new and a lot to deal with, along with the standard issue commitments life brings. The next step is to implement the housekeeping protocol for taking medications and diarise any improvements or hiccups for a few days. When do they happen? Before my next dose? By how many minutes? As forensic as this sounds, these data points are crucial for ensuring that I reach the elusive medication sweet spot sooner rather than later.

The following week, I schedule a call with Lisa to share my progress. When Dr Sweeney returns I do likewise, confident that I can supply more granular information to assist on my health journey. Every Parkinson's experience is unique, which means medication and lifestyle changes must also be customised. You see, I told you PD was a diva.

As a woman in perimenopause, this makes things extra challenging as both conditions share similar symptoms, including brain fog, fatigue and anxiety. This means I must be one step ahead, always guessing its next move. I begin to wonder if I should start hormone replacement therapy. Not only would it ease those awful night sweats, it would sort out my wonky cycle. This way, I can pinpoint when I ovulate and get further clarity with any symptom flare ups.

"That all sounds incredibly demanding," people say to me.

"Perhaps," I reply, "but show me the alternative."

CHAPTER FOUR

Headlines

I'm coming out

July 2022

I'M NOT ONE TO turn down a social occasion. Although a homebody at heart, I love a reason (any reason) to dress up, especially if it involves bubbly and a few fancy appetizers. As a single person, I'm quite used to walking into a party by myself. It doesn't bother me. Chat is my social currency, one which I trade with ease. Should the exchange rate fall or remain flat, I will simply follow the canapés. They never let me down.

Now, things are different. Despite feeling better, I'm not ready to make a post-COVID entrance with Parkinson's as my plus one. Not yet anyway. I need time to feel more comfortable in my body and to accept that this may be my best version of best. I need time, at the very least, to be OK with that.

And so, I sideline invitations to industry events and big mixers – anything out of my comfort zone that might increase stress levels and activate my tremor or dyskinesia. I also turn down hosting a charity event. Even with a headset instead of a handheld microphone, I can't risk having my shakes mistaken for nerves. Unless it's an intimate gathering of close friends and family, my RSVP is 'no'.

Like it or not, visibility is important as a freelancer. Staying front of mind is strengthened by being seen, which is a delicate balancing act in itself. Show up at every junket and you lack credibility; attend too few and no one remembers your name. While my heart tells me to stay put, my head wants to remind people that I haven't fallen off the grid.

Time may be a depreciating asset, but timing is far more important as it determines the value of our efforts. If I act out of a place of lack, that's exactly what I'll get. Slow and steady – that's the pace. Everything in due course.

* * *

Change and time have a unique relationship: where there is an abundance of one, often there is a lack of the other. Somewhere in the middle you'll find a leap of faith – a bridge to the future. Do you take it? If you do, everything changes, but how remains to be seen.

Today is the day that changes everything: the day Vickie, my features director, commissions me to write a special piece for the *Irish Examiner*. It's the day I say "yes" to opening up about my diagnosis, coming out of the medical closet and showing what Parkinson's looks like. I don't know just how important today is or the extent to which it will change my life. Maybe this is a good thing. Still, I know this is big – bigger than me. It's more than just an article on how I live with Parkinson's; it's my way of getting ahead of it and taking control of the narrative. Parkinson's might be the main character, but I am the author. I must not forget this.

Meanwhile, this is the first time my story will go beyond my immediate circle, or on Instagram, for that matter. Back in April, I posted an image of a red tulip (the official Parkinson's emblem) on my grid to mark Parkinson's Awareness Week, along with a few lesser-known facts, one being that I have the disease. My 5,000 or so followers were unbelievably supportive, which gave me the confidence to show up more authentically. So, in June, I put together some educational reels on TikTok and Instagram, sharing how I handle Parkinson's and the unexpected things I deal with on my health journey. I wanted to show others you can live well, however challenging, with Parkinson's. Pity parties aren't my scene. I neither host them nor do I attend them. Typically, there's only one person there, and the snacks are never that great. Don't get me started on the music.

Coming out is not easy. With Parkinson's, there's a lot of baggage, like social stigma, assumptions based on stereotypes and emotional fallout in the forms of anxiety and depression. Disclosing a diagnosis can be career-threatening, and for those who hold caretaking responsibilities, it can be a source of huge stress. Don't get me wrong. For the most part, people will surprise you with their generosity of spirit. Nonetheless, don't be taken aback if someone you least expect doesn't react quite as generously. You quickly learn who your friends are.

I trust Vickie though, and I know she has my back. She gives me plenty of lead time and lets me look at the feature layout before going to print, offering me the power to veto up to the final hour. Not that I do.

There is no point in being on this journey if I'm not willing to share it; no point complaining that Parkinson's needs a makeover if I won't show my face; no point in this pointless disease unless I expose my soft underbelly. I'm privileged to have this platform – a safe space, however vast, in which to share my experience. If I can positively affect one person by doing so, I'll have done my job.

And so, I write 1,600 words, most of them in one sitting, which indicates that I'm on the right track – a flow state, if you will. The content is deeply personal, but I don't feel exposed. Instead, I feel grounded, like I finally own my story. There's immense strength in vulnerability. It's the connective tissue that binds the human experience, regardless of our life paths. If I'm going to fight Parkinson's, this is my weapon of choice.

Vickie tells me the feature will run as the cover story of *Weekend* magazine on August 27th – the same day as my mom's 80th birthday. Although this will be my 11th front cover with the paper, it may as well be my first. Everyone in Munster reads the *Irish Examiner*. It's practically sacrilegious not to. It might be a national broadsheet, but its roots are in the Rebel County – *pure Cork, like*. This level of visibility requires a carefully executed glam strategy. Vulnerability might be my weapon of choice, but so is Miki – a much-loved colleague, fashion photographer and all-star magic maker. Miki's gift is making you feel like you're not getting your photo taken or that you haven't, for that matter, been co-opted into some weird hostage situation, forced to smile as your face bears the strain of terror. I arrange for him to take the pictures in my apartment. This is my sanctuary – the place where I feel most comfortable and at home. He positions the Eames chair – Andy's favourite – at the best angle to catch the late afternoon light, while I give one final check to my outfit: a forest-green asymmetric top and matching wide-leg trousers. As I get situated in my first pose, the sunlight streams from the southwest through the floor-to-ceiling windows, like a golden hour from the gods.

Twenty-three degrees Celsius with blue skies – I couldn't have asked for a better day. Apart from a 30-minute altercation with false eyelashes and fiddly earring backings that morning, which I share for laughs on Instagram, everything goes smoothly. The pictures are natural, glowing and they feel like me – my best version of best.

I catch up with Neil over the phone that evening, entertaining him with my Tremor versus Earrings fight to the death. "I think my future is in clip-ons," I reveal, massaging one of my sore lobes.

Neil belly-laughs. "We need an Instagram story of you removing one so you can answer the landline at Southfork – with a tumbler of vodka."

"Poor Sue Ellen," I lament. "She never quite got over her second husband, Dusty, leaving her to become a rodeo cowboy."

"All joking aside," he insists, "I'm glad you went with the bougie two-piece. If anything says, 'I'm no victim,' it's a large dose of *Dallas*-inspired glamour."

Shifting tone, Neil segues from comic banter to some worrying news. Andy is very stressed. He's having trouble with his right leg, including a recent fall at work. While he's waiting for an emergency appointment with a neurologist, his mind is going to dark places – the worst-case scenario. Andy isn't one to catastrophise or jump to conclusions, which gives us pause, even if we don't admit to it. Maybe he knows something we don't – a gut feeling. It seems trite to tell him he has our unconditional support when we can't do anything, all of us stuck in a holding pattern, hoping for the best. Hope might be a fool's medicine, but that's all we have until we know more. Until then, we wait.

August 2022

It's dark. Where the hell am I? Panicked, I bolt upright in bed, hitting the back of my head against the stippled roof.

Is this a child's room? A rowdy gang of expletives look for a hasty exit. I tighten security, aware the others are still asleep, and I get my bearings while I come around. The faint sound of seagulls and waves reminds me I'm on Inishbofin. Of course. This is the cottage my sister rented for Mom's eightieth birthday weekend (a.k.a. 'Mom Fest'). Why, at six feet tall, I choose to sleep in the loft is anyone's guess. Remaining crouched, I search around in the semi-light for a robe and slippers, and I carefully descend the wooden ladder to make some coffee and check my messages before everyone else wakes up.

Knowing that today would be a big day, I left the pub early last night. I need to be more mindful of my energy levels these days. I'm also a lightweight. Let's not gloss over that fact. Two glasses of wine and I'm tipsy. Three glasses and you may as well pre-book an ambulance. From what I understand, shots, dancing and traditional music made an appearance after my departure, so I don't expect to see the others too soon.

First things first, I call Mom to say happy birthday and tell her that I'll be over to her place once I have breakfast.

Ping. Maureen texts me on her way to catch the midday boat to Inishbofin. *I picked up three copies of the* Examiner *in Galway. Do you need more?*

Another ping. It's Julie. *I got five copies. You look stunning!*

Attached are two snapshots: the front cover of the *Irish Examiner* and one of *Weekend* magazine. The headline reads "Annmarie O'Connor on the diagnosis that changed her life".

Ping. It's Vickie asking how I am and letting me know that the online feature is already clocking up a considerable number of views. She reckons it will be the most-read story by afternoon.

This is a lot to absorb, especially with no caffeine in my system, which I remedy immediately. When I open Instagram on my phone, I notice a few hundred new followers and dozens of messages from well-wishers who have read the feature. I'm taken aback. My email inbox looks similar. Total strangers offering support, prayers and encouragement – many of them with a personal experience of Parkinson's or a family member with the disease.

"Articles like yours are so important. It's easy to feel alone with things like this," writes one person.

"Your words filled the jigsaw piece I needed," says another.

I spot a message from one of my colleagues: "I feel like all of your work to date has been leading up to what you are going to do – the world is your stage, and it is in your vulnerability that the greatest power lies."

This warms my heart. I promise myself to respond to these messages later this afternoon, before we head to dinner. In the meantime, I post a link to the feature on my Instagram Feed and Stories before I mute the app notifications on my phone, butter two pieces of sourdough toast and get dressed.

I take the scenic route along the East End strand towards Cloonamore. Stepping over wigs of reddish seaweed and sandcastles left by razor clams, I remember this is where I learned to walk. A bit of a late bloomer, I was 15 months old before I trusted myself to put one foot in front of the other. Perfectly capable of standing on my own two feet, I was too afraid to take it to the next level, always holding onto a banister or railing before cautiously dropping to my knees and crawling.

When I did let go, it was to head towards the familiar sound of my father's voice as he arrived at the gable door of Nana's house. Working full time as a correction officer at the Bronx House of Detention, he couldn't join Mom and us girls until later that summer. According to island lore, I didn't just walk, I ran.

Breaking my reverie, I look out at the expanse of seawater and spot a rubber-clad head breaching the stillness. It's Mags who, to no one's surprise, is having her morning dip, which will be followed by a sneaky swim this afternoon and, if she can swing it, another one before we head to Murray's for dinner. I wave and she bobs. We'll catch up later, no doubt. Rumour has it that Mags has a Mom Fest spreadsheet for the next few days. Why am I not surprised?

With the strand behind me, I make my way up the mountain path, past the lavender and blackberry verges, my sister Kate's organic vegetable tunnel and her donkey Darwin's old stomping ground. Fuchsia honeysuckles jut from the stone walls, offering their nectar to anyone willing to encounter an end-of-summer wasp. As I negotiate the last hill before reaching Mom's back gate, I think of Nana and Mom – both ahead of their time – teaching us when to pick the berries and how to release honey from the flower stem. Mini foragers in the making, our palms were mostly covered in red sticky petals and purple juice, but that was half the fun.

* * *

Later, I'm sitting in my mother's green armchair with Rosie the pug on my lap, snoring for all she's worth. RTÉ Radio 1 plays on the kitchen stereo while crosscurrents of conversation intersect between Mom and an incoming stream of daughters, partners and grandchildren. The cacophony is familial and fun, but probably not the best place to answer a phone call, I think, as I spot an unknown Dublin number flashing on my screen.

I deposit Rosie beside Patricia and excuse the interruption, taking my business outside.

Much to my surprise, it's a producer from the *Brendan O'Connor* radio show. Having read my Parkinson's story in the *Irish Examiner*, she invites me to be a guest on the programme in early September. Naturally, I say yes, and we arrange to firm up details after the weekend. Before returning inside to share my good news, I quickly check my Instagram and email. Hundreds more direct messages, reposts and comments join the growing contingent. In an age of online feuds and internet trolls, I'm humbled by the response and encouraged by the kindness of people. From invitations to join support groups to individuals offering an ear or advice whenever I need it, it reminds me that once shared, any experience is a collective one. No one is alone.

A text message appears from Vickie: *Just checking in to see how you are. You must have had a huge response. The piece is trending at number one on today's most-read articles. The numbers are really high. You should be proud of yourself. You are helping so many people.*

Mom will be so thrilled to hear this, but I'm conscious that this is her big day. I want to be present for her, so I put my calls on silent, which upon reflection, is pointless; I challenge anyone to hear themselves think over the collective volume of our voices. We're a garrulous lot.

There is so much happening for Mom Fest, from unveiling Patricia's elaborate birthday cake at dinner to my video tribute later this evening, and Maureen's enormous photo collage – the centrepiece at tomorrow's party in The Galley. Mom isn't one for big displays and is a person who, generally, likes her own company, but she's coming out this weekend in a big way. She deserves the spotlight.

At 17 years old, she moved to New York to work, just like her sister had done four years prior, with both of them sending money home to Ireland. After my father's death, she did the work of two people, despite making the money of one and having to look after five. A multi-hyphenate grafter, she decorated cakes, altered clothes, baked brown bread and apple tarts and ran a guesthouse. The odds weren't stacked in her favour, but she made it look easy despite the sacrifices. I have always been amazed at her ability to create something from nothing – a sleight of hand mastered by few. An impeccable dressmaker, she made our special wardrobe pieces from Vogue and Butterick patterns. "It wasn't off the wind she caught it," as the old Irish saying goes. Her father, a tailor, could chalk up a suit without using a measuring tape. Not to mention Nana, who'd get the measure of you in two seconds flat.

Trips to the fabric store were not uncommon in our childhood, sorting through bolts of velvet, tweed and wool while learning about finishing touches like decent zippers and buttons. Not one to confuse value and cost, she taught me about capsule dressing, mastering the art of good basics and how to have more with less – life skills that inform my world to this day. She didn't just meet our needs; she made us feel abundant. That alone is worth celebrating.

* * *

I leave Mom's house a bit earlier so I can walk the beach and get my emotional bearings, conscious that anxiety worsens my tremor. Today is not your average news day, that's for sure. Despite the outpouring of support, the impact of this level of attention feels overwhelming. Not one to immediately process things, I need to ground myself before opening my phone again. With my face breeze-bound, I inhale and receive the moment as my soft, wet steps leave their marks in the sand.

By the time I reach the cottage, I realise I'm the only one there. In the interests of sheer vanity, this also serves me well. I'm impossibly slow at getting ready, especially when it comes to styling my hair. I could ask one of the kids or my sisters to help, but I don't want to be a pain. Operating curling tongs at 200 degrees Celsius in an attic room is asking for trouble, as I crouch like a hobbit to make sure not to hit the wand off the stippled ceiling. When my aching arms tell me to leave well enough alone, I stop and drop, put on my favourite vintage dress and carry my espadrille wedges down the ladder. There will be no sprained ankles or trips to the nurse this weekend, thanks very much.

A dry robe with wet paraphernalia in hand appears at the Dutch door, opening the latch from the inside.

"Hey, Mags. We missed you at Mom's. How was the water?"

"Fantastic. I popped up to see her while you were showering. She told me your good news. I'm dying to hear about the *Brendan O'Connor Show*. Give me one second . . ."

Her voice tails off briefly as she hangs wetsuits on the clothesline and shakes out sandy towels. For the record, Margaret, a die-hard rugby fan, would leave an Ireland vs All Blacks final on the telly with a try and two minutes hanging in the balance to hang laundry on a fine day, such is her commitment to the cause.

"That was my second swim." She closes the back door on her confession before disappearing into the laundry room and emerging with the drying basket. "I thought I'd have time for another, but we need to be at Murray's by six this evening and . . ."

"It's not on the spreadsheet!" I cry out, clutching my invisible pearls.

Margaret feigns a laugh, tucking damp tendrils of hair behind her ear – a tick that manifests when she feels under pressure. "I was going to make coffee, but I better stop faffing and hit the shower. Before I do . . ." She locates her phone and reading glasses on the kitchen table beside the three copies of today's paper. "Come here. I want you to look at something." Tapping the 6.7-inch OLED screen in her hand, she shows me a dozen or so well-wishes, text messages and DMs from her friends about today's Parkinson's feature.

Maureen arrives from Mom's and joins our mini summit. "Excuse this disaster," she apologises, brandishing her damaged phone, which landed on the kitchen floor last week in an ill-timed leap of fate. "I put up your post on Facebook about an hour ago. Just look at the response!" Words such as *brave, inspiring, warrior* and *insightful* fill the cracks in the screen. It feels like a case of mistaken identity. I'm the person who is petrified of heights, who dreads making bad decisions, and who, categorically, will not pass a magpie without waving. Let's not get started on my fear of the future, which keeps me awake at night. Word to the wise: never consult an online pension calculator before bed. Brave? Hardly.

"In all honesty, we couldn't be prouder of you, especially Mom," Margaret beams before excusing herself to freshen up. Tired of standing, Maureen and I take a seat on the sofa across from the stone fireplace. Exhaling in tandem, we pause. I take my phone notifications off silent.

"How are you feeling about everything?" Maureen hooks her forearm around mine, afraid I'll be swept away.

"Honestly, I didn't expect this reaction. It's humbling but hard to get my head around. It feels like I won an award I didn't deserve. You know?"

She gives me an incredulous head tilt. "That's very modest of you but a bit off base. Why else would your phone be blowing up?"

Ping. Ping. Ping. Ping.

Spawning notifications, multiple missed calls and texts, not to mention a serpentine list of unanswered emails, validate her claim. I tentatively swipe my screen and scroll, scroll, scroll. My finger keeps scrolling, searching for completion.

Maureen makes room for awe. "Moments like these are rare, so don't be afraid to take it all in. And to think, we still have tonight and tomorrow to enjoy."

Just then, two of the kids return from the shops with milk and extra cereal for the morning. Laughing, messing, Spotify playlists and high-pitched hair dryers play together. Kate will be here soon to bring the first carful of revellers to Murray's. This is the sound of family. Mom Fest is in full swing.

* * *

The next day, Maureen and I leave The Galley earlier than the others to catch the one o'clock boat, as we both have work the following morning. I got the part-time copyediting role. The HR manager and I agree to give it two months to see if it's a good fit for both parties. This sounds fair, and frankly, I am grateful for the wiggle room.

Even though my symptoms are more manageable of late, the redux of painful, restless legs over the past few nights makes me anxious. I tell myself it's from sleeping in a smaller bed than usual, but I know I'm only fooling myself. By the time I get home to Cork, it's 8 p.m. I'm spent. I barely have the energy to unpack and get cleaned up before I text the family group chat and go to bed. The following day, life picks up pace and the lingering residue of fatigue gives way to exciting prospects and possibilities. Every email I open feels like I'm a game show contestant on a winning streak.

A booker from *The Tommy Tiernan Show* contacts me to gauge my interest in being an upcoming guest on the programme. I'm gobsmacked. As a journalist, I am such a fan, and I love the premise of interviewing guests without any preparation or knowledge of who will be joining Tommy until they meet in studio. As a classic over-preparer, that would be my nightmare, which makes it so compelling.

I also get word that my slot with Brendan O'Connor is scheduled for this Saturday. Lisa, the Parkinson's Ireland specialist nurse, contacts me to share the impact of my *Irish Examiner* story on the number of calls to the charity's hotline.

"The response has been fantastic," she writes. "It has given those people I have spoken to a nudge and a lift, which is so positive. I look forward to speaking to more who may be encouraged to reach out."

Then comes an email from Dr Sweeney. A colleague of his who attended the Movement Disorder Society meeting in Madrid said that my article was mentioned in one of the plenary sessions by the keynote speaker, Professor Susan Fox. Any minute now, Oprah is going to tell me I won a car.

It's easy to feel optimistic when the news is this good. Nonetheless, the pragmatist in me demands I focus on what's in front of me. And so, I do. This time, I'm not holding a banister. This time, I'm running.

* * *

Sitting in a radio studio alone at RTÉ Cork, I wait to be patched into the *Brendan O'Connor Show*. A producer tests my microphone and tells me it'll be another few minutes, just after the news. I'm nervous, although I shouldn't be. Fourteen years as a fashion contributor on various radio programmes is no mean feat. This is different. My vulnerability is getting airtime. The show is live with no delete button. Should I make a mistake, I can't take it back. *But there are no mistakes*, I remind myself. *This is your story. Tell it with candour. That's all you need to do.*

When I am given the floor to share my personal history, I lead with my heart. Much in the same way as I did in the *Irish Examiner*, I detail my Parkinson's journey from symptoms to diagnosis, explaining how I now live and work with the disorder in the face of my strict day-to-day routine.

"Does this define your life now?" Brendan asks, intrigued by my scrupulous medication regimen and lifestyle changes. *What a good question.* I nod my head in appreciation, so used to third parties with no lived experience or medical qualifications telling me how Parkinson's works.

"People have said to me, 'Look, Parkinson's won't define your life.' I've corrected them and said, 'No, but it's part of my life.' As much as I have brown eyes, I am six-foot tall and I work as a writer, I also have Parkinson's disease," I explain. "Thus, that determines what I do and how I move through the world. But it's not the end of the world."

As for the future? I tell him I see it as an ellipsis. For every heartening story of a person with Parkinson's running a marathon, another is having their skull drilled for deep brain stimulation therapy where a battery-operated remote is inserted adjacent to their collarbone to control motor symptoms. "It's the kind of thief that can steal your dignity and your identity if you let it. You can be aware of it without making allowances for its sneaky behaviour," I add.

I highlight helpful resources in Ireland for those diagnosed, their families and carers. We say goodbye and thank you, and the red button turns off, signalling I can remove my headset. The producer sees me out, and I walk down Father Matthew Street feeling that bit lighter, my sleeveless arms befitting the warm September breeze. *It's not the end of the world. I can live with this.* Taking my phone off airplane mode, I realise why. So many people support me. Texts, missed calls and Instagram DMs. Once I have the chance to catch my breath and read the messages, I am stunned at how many people keep their diagnosis quiet, silenced by shame or apprehension.

As I said to Brendan about my medical coming out, "Nothing grows in the darkness. So, if we can shed a bit of light on this disease, which is so evasive, people will begin to understand it, not fear it." After all, vulnerability and fear can't co-exist; one will always cancel the other out. I turn the corner towards South Mall and step onto the sun-dappled footpath. My face gravitates skyward, seeking out the light.

This is who I am. I have Parkinson's. There's no reason to hide.

CHAPTER FIVE

Grief

Goodbye, old life

August 2022

EXCUSE ME FOR THE interruption. Grief is here. I admit it. There's never a suitable time for her to drop by: grief doesn't make plans, she never calls in advance, she won't read the room. Instead, she shows up at the most inopportune moments, demanding your attention and giving little in return.

Sometimes grief plays the long game, creating a false sense of security before arriving, unannounced but not unfamiliar – like today. This is not our first meeting and probably not our last. Still, it doesn't make it any easier. What puts things into perspective is understanding how I know her so well. Correction: how *we* know her so well. My family is no stranger to grief, yet they manage to keep their distance. With a history of hard knocks and sudden losses, callused hands and worried minds, grief is a privilege open to others – not to us. There simply isn't room for crying when life falls apart. Who has the time? Besides, emotions are liquid and hard to contain. It's best we keep eyes dry and chins up. For now, anyway. Sooner or later, grief gets her way as we scream into the wind and rain, allowing tears to lose their identity, our hearts cursing the tide.

To understand me and my story better, allow me to take you back in time to the moments that changed my life and the lives of the women before me, our shared tragedies and the history that binds us. It might go some way to explain my complicated relationship with grief and its role in my Parkinson's journey.

* * *

Christmas Day, 1977: At the hospital, they administer the last rites, turn off the machines and pronounce the time of death shortly after 7 p.m. Just like that. Gone. Patricia wakes me up the following morning to tell me Daddy died. I turn over and go back to sleep, too young, at four years old, to grasp the permanence of death. My mother and sisters wear black as the trumpets play "Taps" and a rifle performs the three-volley salute, while I stay home with a family friend and play alone.

Weeks go by and the familiar absence grows. People lower their voices and spell out his name in my presence as if his death is a secret yet to be revealed. I feel sad but hopeful that God will let him come home. Only He doesn't. Instead of my father, we have an American flag folded in the shape of a triangle from the police department. Mom keeps it with the Waterford crystal and the good tableware in the dining room curio cabinet. I wonder why it's there and where Daddy is now as I spend my days watching clouds, mistaking them for Heaven. We fly to Ireland that summer, and I ask my mother if the pilot might stop the plane so that we can visit Daddy. It takes a year before I understand what dead means, courtesy of a school bully. Daddy's brain burst and he is not coming home. Stop waiting.

1978: Close to my birthday, a few months after my father died, I make the declaration that I am not turning five. I don't want to get older. I don't want a communion. I certainly don't want to get married. I plan on staying four forever. This is my happily ever after. When Mom tries to explain that life goes on and I will, indeed, grow up, I exhibit a pointless act of defiance as if throwing a tantrum will stop time. I want things to stay as they are. No more change. I want the status quo.

1979: It's Father's Day and we are making cards in school. My first-grade teacher mocks me openly in front of the class. "Annmarie can't make a card for Father's Day. Annmarie doesn't have a father." Dead. It's the bully all over again. I feel small. A knot forms in my throat, tightening and tightening. It hurts.

1980: We pass the cannon at Battery Park, where the men play chess, which tells me we've left Long Island behind. Shortly, we'll climb the tiled stairs to Grandma's fourth-floor walk-up on Eighth Avenue, guided by the familiar scent of baked ham. I love visiting her apartment. She always has Dr Pepper cola in her fridge, dinner in the oven, and she can make an apple pie materialise at will. With the sash window open to cool down the kitchen, you can feel the muggy city breath do its best. I ask to see her photo album – a heavy tome covered in plastic wrapping, like the covering on her sofa and carpet. Filled with sepia-toned Polaroids of Daddy and Uncle Johnny as little boys, Grandma and Poppy at Coney Island, my aunts in their marching band outfits, I can't help but smile. Daddy's side of the family is where I get my height, people say, especially my long fingers and feet.

"A big house needs a big foundation," Grandma says. "Otherwise, it will topple over." Even though I spend most of my time looking at pictures of my father, there are, I notice, none of Grandma as a young girl. As a kid, I know the age-appropriate version of how she moved to America, which, along with Dad's passing, informs my childhood fear of Mom dying and me being taken away.

Grandma's widowed and physically unwell father had a difficult time managing his County Kerry farm and five young children. When a cousin from America came to visit, a proposal was made that saw Grandma, aged seven, and her five-year-old brother make the three-week boat journey from Cobh in Cork to New York. Placed in steerage with this blood stranger for company, the pair were being taken to 'visit' family in America, or so they were told. Upon arrival, the siblings, now free from the stench of vomit and faeces of the boat, were separated and forced to work for relatives in different states. Her brother kept an 80-year-old aunt company in Boston while Grandma looked after the 10 children of the blood stranger's daughter in a suburb of Connecticut. Grandma never spoke much about this part of her life, but she did tell my aunt that some nights she would be up as late as 11 p.m. folding diapers and had yet to start her homework. At 18 years old, she moved in with her sister in Queens, an emigrant by choice, not by cull, and later married a Kerryman, whom she met at a St Patrick's Day dance.

1985: Before we leave America, Grandma brings Mom, the twins and me on a day trip around Manhattan. We ride the F train from 8th Avenue Station to 34th Street and Herald Square and go to the observation deck on the 102nd floor of the Empire State Building. Here, we pick out our favourite skyscrapers and try to locate Grandma's apartment in the distance. Later, we walk through Times Square and take the Staten Island Ferry across New York Harbour. Grandma points out Ellis Island. This is where the RMS *Samaria* from Cobh was due to dock on 13th November 1922 – the day she arrived in America. She doesn't tell me this, nor do I know at the time that the ship rerouted to Boston, where she and her brother were separated. I know the age-appropriate story of Irish immigrants arriving here to find work and new opportunities, not where young girls are sent to do unpaid labour in the Land of the Free. I wave at the Statue of Liberty, unable to see the empty promises etched in her eyes, not knowing what goodbye would mean as we emigrate in reverse.

1985: I am 12 years old when we move to Ireland. The Yanks, they call us. The widow with five girls in the big house. Divorced. Definitely divorced. A guest house, or so the rumours say. They go to mass. Sunday mornings. A divorced woman with five girls at mass. Imagine.

Knock, knock. Mom answers the door. It's the head of a local women's group bearing an apology dressed as an invitation.

"We didn't realise you were a widow." A silly mistake, really. It could happen to anyone, or so they think.

"Now, dear, if I wasn't good enough for you then, I'm certainly not good enough for you now. Good day." Door closed.

Mistaken identity – it's a common trope with us. "That accent's not from here," you hear them say, warming up to, "Do you consider yourself more American or Irish?" Armed with PC answers, I am a cross-cultural diplomat far too young to be auditioning for Miss World. "It must have been hard on you, the move," they say, priming me for a sob story. *No father. One of five. Mother keeps to herself.* Like Mom, I don't fall for it. More mind-your-own-business-style answers follow.

The truth is the move felt sudden and out of my control. The decision was made for me: a brave one, the right one, but not my one. Still, I refuse to let people pity me like they did when my father died. Pity is superior and stingy: an empty-handed gesture that offers nothing to the recipient. The first grade taught me that.

Mom urges me to own my height. "Nothing is worse than a tall girl who slouches." She puts books on my head and two-inch heels on my feet. "Take up space," she tells me. "Be seen."

I need to. School is different: uniforms and the smell of damp milk palettes replace the morning flag salute and popularity wars. My accent gets the most attention: the sniggering, the poor attempts at mockery.

"Go back to America," some say.

"One day," I retort. "Or any day, for that matter. I have two passports. Tell me, when is that Green Card lottery again?"

Now, I stand tall. I stand up for myself. The casual bullying stops and respect fills the void. I talk about America like I do about Dad – in the past tense.

1989: Grief arrives and apologises for the delay. I am 16 when we meet again. The emotional numbing cream wears off, and I feel pain once more after the moment that altered the course of my life. It's a relief. I can finally cry.

Those childhood Sundays in America when we would visit the cemetery, trying to find Daddy's grave among the identical rows of numbered headstones – those were hard. Section A, near the little tree. Mom could never seem to find him despite us visiting every month. Upset, no doubt, because she keeps losing him. After saying the "Our Father" prayer together, I would watch Mom and the girls struggle to remain composed, wiping errant tears out of sight. Despite trying my best, I couldn't find the same release for my emptiness. After all, you can't grieve something you never had, and in the pecking order, I am thought to have the least collateral damage – by others, that is. The same ones that spell out his name. *Lucky to be so young. Lucky not to remember.* They would say it, hint it, think it. *That* I know.

It's as if grief intuits that I am better equipped to process the shock of loss as a teenager. I start asking questions, second-guessing if my memories are inherited or authentically mine. Maybe the others are right. Maybe I was too young. My mother cottons on to grief's MO and takes me out of school for a week – a kindness for which I'll always be grateful. She listens as I talk. We occupy the kitchen with photo albums and colourful anecdotes. Day by day, we speak Dad into the present with precious rescue breaths, world-building and validating moments as valuable assets that belong to me alone. We are not a family who comes from money, but what my mother helps accrue over those few days pays dividends in peace and clarity. Before long, healing occurs and freshly pink scar tissue forms.

Grief's late arrival, although welcome, comes with baggage. There's only so much you can unpack, especially when life shows you so little. I don't know it then, but I am afraid: afraid to be a *burden*, afraid people will leave if they get too close, afraid to give too much of myself – afraid to love.

1997: I learn very quickly that it isn't safe to have what I want. I spend my mid-twenties and most of my thirties playing adjacent to my desires and needs. I live on the sidelines, accepting pointless jobs instead of pursuing my passion, running away from emotionally available relationships, desperate not to be vulnerable. I fear stepping into my power and going after what I want, lest it is taken away. I fear rejection – a second death.

2021: These fears remain hidden in plain sight until my Parkinson's diagnosis in December. If you look closely enough, you can catch their shadows. They're everywhere and nowhere at once. Despite my whole life changing in an instant, I don't see Parkinson's as something to grieve, not yet anyway. Just like my four-year-old self, I'm not sure what I have lost. I should be angry at this careless twist of fate – the destabilising uncertainty of knowing my body and mind will deteriorate but not knowing when. Instead, I attach my old life to machines, despite time of death being called – waiting for normalcy to return. It never does.

What I don't realise is how Parkinson's will rattle me, so much so that it will awaken the genetic script within, the one made of sea salt and grit. It will activate my name, Annmarie, meaning 'grace' and 'rebelliousness'. First, it needs to break me. One day this will happen. That is certain.

I am not certain, however, not certain of my future, or of my choices. Afraid I am travelling in the wrong direction once more, I look for guidance. It's no surprise to me that when I receive an audio reading from a psychic medium, it's the spirit of my Nana, my maternal grandmother from Inishbofin, who comes through. I am honoured.

My mother always said, "She wouldn't call the Queen her aunt," so I accept Nana's visit with a mental curtsy. Everyone knew who the boss lady was on the East End of Inishbofin, and her name was Catherine O'Toole.

Much like Grandma, Nana's early years were punctuated by tragedy. At age 10, she lost her mother. Seven years later, her father, a fish buyer, died in the Cleggan Disaster – an unexpected hurricane that resulted in the death of 45 fishermen off the coast of Galway. Having hurt his foot, her father wasn't due to go to sea that evening but, at the last minute, he went in place of a sick crewman. His body was found washed up on the Claddaghduff shoreline – according to lore, with a slipper on one foot and a boot on the other. His was the only body to be found. Nana, now 17, became head of her household: mother and father, as well as sister. She cooked, cleaned and knitted Aran sweaters for Stanleys in Clifden to put her five siblings through school. Neither a saint nor a martyr, Nana was a rebel. On the run from Cromwell, her ancestors fled County Wicklow, making Clifden and the island of Inishturk (meaning 'wild boar') their homes. At eight months pregnant, she walked five miles there and back to dry turf at Westquarter

Mountain. Although not one to start anything, you could be guaranteed she'd finish it, including an altercation with a spirit that allegedly haunted her marital home, until she told it off with words that would make a sailor blush. Afraid? Well, I imagine the ghost was.

Not unlike my paternal grandmother and my mother, her bravery and fortitude in the presence of indescribable odds act as my inner compass, as does her refusal to play the victim. Perspective is a necessary lens. Without it, we remain at sea, adrift of our experiences and our choices. So long as I listen, I can't go too far wrong.

January 2023: The medium sends me the pre-recorded reading via WhatsApp. A bit like Wi-Fi, she can tune into a person's frequency remotely to make a connection. Impressed with the efficiency, I press play and get cosy on my comfy chair. Nana shows her a clear outline of a glass heart with a gold centre – fragile but strong. I protect it from those who try getting close. And no one does. It is a defence mechanism, and I am resolute, or so Nana insists. *Afraid to love. Afraid to be a burden.* I'm beginning to think my Google Assistant is a portal to the other side. It's not the Russians listening; it's my Irish granny.

Nana tells me to let go of my old identity, my protective shields and my determination to soldier through this independently. Reach out; ask for help; be vulnerable. *She can be very insistent.* I can tell this from the medium's tone, who, I imagine, is being badgered by a five-foot-five woman with white curly hair.

As the medium reminds me that our family has come through terrible times together before, I remember the graveyard: section A near the little tree, the collective tears and me on the outside looking in – waiting. When she uses the word 'grief', Nana's reputation as a straight shooter with no time for nonsense jolts me into awareness.

I am not OK. This is not OK. I know what's next. It's time to meet grief again. There's no avoiding it.

Nana, of course, is right.

* * *

Grief calls by when I least expect it. She tries the door handle and lets herself in. I thought I locked it, but her smile says otherwise. Increasingly, she stays longer and longer, refusing to leave despite me having things to do. At times, she insists on sleeping over, keeping me awake at night.

Then, one day, she strikes me suddenly and without provocation. I am scrolling casually through videos on my phone when a voiceover says, "With Parkinson's, we manage the symptoms, not treat the disease. It is progressive, incurable and will only get worse."

Despite knowing this in my head, I haven't felt it in my heart. The glass case breaks and I begin to cry. The kind of crying that leaves you spent and takes you for all you've got. The kind that washes over you like so many waves, catching you in a rip curl and spitting you back out on the shore. The kind that stains your cheeks to cleanse your heart. The kind that heals.

And we all need healing, whatever our wounds. We can't accept what is until we mourn what was, nor can we foster faith in what will be. Everything is connected: past, present and future. There is no skipping steps, not without consequences. Trust me, the universe is always watching.

I don't see grief as much anymore, but I won't be so surprised the next time she lets herself in. She always does. Who knows? I might even leave the key under the mat.

CHAPTER SIX

Rebel Yell

Anger is an energy

September 2022

"The day Parkinson's comes for my writing ability: I will be waiting. Mark my words: There will be one hell of a fight."

That is how my *Irish Examiner* feature ends, with me throwing the proverbial gauntlet.

Not one to waste time, Parkinson's calls dibs on my most precious asset. Every day, my tremor increases and my fingers stiffen, making it harder to type. Work becomes slow and uncomfortable despite my best efforts. Hand stretches and warm compresses – nothing gets results.

Mom calls me stoic. "Annmarie accepts the hand she's been dealt," she tells others. "She just gets on with it." Not anymore. I'm tired. Tired of asking for deadline extensions. Tired of saying no to incoming work I'm not fit to complete. Tired of being tired.

Now, I must make good on my promise – one hell of a fight. To look at me, I'm no contender, but I have patience, stubbornness and tenacity on my side, not to mention some displaced hormonal rage. Plus, I'm not one to pull any punches. There's too much to lose. Not only is my livelihood at stake, so is the life I created for myself, the life I love. Give up? I'm just getting started. That's not to say I'll win. But I will fight – that's guaranteed. Do your best, Parkinson's. I'm ready.

* * *

The following week, I'm at my desk trying to finish a piece of online copy. The pads on my fingers land flat against the keyboard. *BANG. BANG. BANG.* It's a stiff day.

What? Shouldn't that be . . .

The paragraph I am working on reads, "My first love has always been riding."

Oh, for god's sake.

I delete the offending word and replace it with 'writing'.

A muffled melody plays from under a stack of notebooks. "Hey, Trish – you're on speakerphone!" I answer before stretching and rubbing my delinquent hands.

"Just thought I'd give you a quick ring while I was in the car. How are things?"

"Oh, you know . . ." Of course, she does. She would, no less. In addition to her super-sensitive nose, Patricia has a weird sixth sense when I'm feeling down. The obvious quaver in my voice doesn't help matters.

"Tell me what's wrong."

"Nothing's wrong," I try to assure her.

Knowing silence enters the chat.

"I'm just so exasperated, Trish. I feel like an invisible bully is taunting my body. If it's not one thing, it's another." After disclosing my recent episode of self-sabotage, much to her amusement, the conversation gets serious.

"The dyskinesia in my left shoulder is back. So is the tremor in my hand and my little finger is so painfully stiff I can barely type. I'm still waking with restless legs every morning, now between 2.30 and 4.30 a.m., but with pains in my toes and ankles too," I explain. "To cap it off, my right leg either feels like it's limping or shaky. Sometimes I can't feel it at all, unlike the ungodly spasms in my right foot." I refresh her memory about dystonia – the pain like an assault from Vecna's telekinetic powers in my right arch, sole and toes that brings me to tears.

"You've got an outpatient appointment soon, don't you?" she asks, reminding me that the 21st is next Wednesday – nearer than I think. "Have you looked into speech-to-text recognition software to help with your articles?"

"Yes, but dictation would be a new skill I'd have to learn on top of learning about Parkinson's, getting used to medication and trying to make a living. It's a lot of change hitting me at once. Also, the copyediting job didn't work out."

"You only started a few weeks ago. What happened?"

"I was way too slow. My fingers were rigid and cramping. Plus, my insomnia made a comeback. If I hadn't quit, I would have been let go, for sure. Thankfully, it was still during my probation period. I just feel embarrassed that my quality of work is slipping. Not to mention, my bank balance. Things are tight and I don't have the feet for OnlyFans."

We start chuckling with no end in sight.

About 15 years ago, on a Greek sun holiday, a woman approached me, unprompted, about my hammer toes. "There's something that can be done about them," she advised while recommending 'a great doctor' at Harley Street Clinic. My feet have remained covered since.

"On a positive note," I continue, "I started cyclical HRT in August which means my monthly cycle is back to every

28 days. I can now confidently discern if a spike in my motor symptoms is due to ovulation or my period. I also get the kickback of reduced night sweats – silver linings and all that."

"Well, there you go. It's OK to feel discouraged. Even if there isn't much you can do about it now, it'll spur you to find a solution—

"The *right* solution," she stresses, "in due course. You'll look back at this as a blip on the radar, I've no doubt."

"Fingers crossed," I say.

* * *

The more I learn about Parkinson's, the less I know and the more confused I become. What I am certain of is that with Parkinson's, there's always a trade-off. At my outpatient meeting with Dr Sweeney, I inform him of my persistent tremor issues. He prescribes an anticholinergic drug used to treat stiffness, tremors, spasms and poor muscle control as an assist to my L-dopa. Cognition problems in the elderly cohort are the main concern, but thankfully, age aside, my mental faculties are sharp – sleepless nights notwithstanding. Otherwise, it is well tolerated. Within two days, a small miracle happens. My tremor, dyskinesia, dystonia and restless legs are gone. Two days later, I am sleeping through the night (the first time in months) without waking up to take an extra tablet. Most of all, my typing is back to being smooth and speedy.

Parkinson's always looks for payback, though, and isn't shy about collecting its debt. The trade-off? I either feel so fatigued that I need to go back to bed or I feel high. The sensation is comparable to an out-of-body experience or coming up from ecstasy in a club. This happens either immediately or 40 to 90 minutes after a dose. What's more, there is no warning. At times, it catches me off guard, like yesterday in the Tesco frozen food aisle or this morning when I couldn't feel my legs. Combine my low threshold for medication with a physical adjustment period of anywhere from four to six weeks and we've got ourselves a problem. You see, I'm being weaned onto the drug and won't be at full tilt for another six days.

How ironic. I finally get my fine motor skills back and I'm too out of it to work. This must be what cosmic spite looks like. Here's the thing: when something isn't good enough, I send it back. I don't let it take up space in my life. The question is, do I see out the habituation period in the hopes the euphoric side effects will level off, or do I give up now and try something else?

* * *

September evenings in Ireland are special. Days retreat with a distinct coolness as the pink sky prepares for dusk. Like an imperfect goodbye, it's beautiful to watch one slip away. And we do, latching on to the final vestige of summer as we walk and talk, just Julie and me.

"It's surreal, Jules. One minute, I'm fine, and the next, I'm completely spaced out." I tell her about my recent unsettling incident on the 220 bus, unaware that it's 5.30 p.m. This means my 5 p.m. dose is now kicking in. "We're travelling along the Douglas Road and as the bus emerges from beneath the overpass, BOOM – my body is warm and tingly, and I start seeing laser beams of light. It's like being inside a rainbow."

At this stage, I start picking up speed both in steps and words per minute as we approach the bottom of Coach Hill. Julie lags, finding it hard to keep up with me as I tackle the vertiginous ascent, talking and talking. God, I can't stop talking.

"Annie, can you slow down a bit?" Julie pants. From the girl who runs Maryborough Hill four times a week, this is damning evidence. I'm wired, there is no denying it. Much of the 'walk' is punctuated by me cantering ahead, telling no one in particular about my dilated pupils and subsequent bouts of full-body fatigue, so much so that we miss the Rochestown sunset – Julie too preoccupied with my euphoric burst and me, well, too high to notice.

The chaotic marathon finishes before the roundabout across from Julie's house. She convinces me to come in for a cup of tea, which I later discover is a concerned and clever ruse to drive me home, even if it is only three minutes away. By the time we're in her car, I'm more subdued.

"I can't keep this up."

"No, I imagine you can't." Julie turns off the ignition as we pause for a beat outside of my apartment.

"What are you going to do, Annie?"

"I'll sort this out," I half-whisper. "Maybe it's a matter of a lower dosage."

"Maybe it is, but I'm worried about the level of decisions you need to make while sleep-deprived, stressed and now strung out."

"Me too," I confess. "It's just heartbreaking to have a miracle in my grasp only to watch it slip away. Part of me wants to hang on a bit longer in the hopes that habituation kicks in, but I don't know if that's practical." Julie's concerned eyebrows say it all.

"I'll look at a more sustainable solution with my consultant tomorrow – whether that's tweaking the dosage or going back to my usual prescription." I nod, approving my choice in real time.

"I think that's smart. Now, go get some sleep," Julie insists as I unlock my seatbelt. "Let me know how you get on during the week. And Annie?"

"What's that?" I ask before closing the passenger door.
"Thanks for saving me a trip to the gym tomorrow."

October 2022

"I can't believe I spent good money on this thing," I mutter, tossing a plastic pill cutter, my latest accessory, into the odds and sods drawer. My oh my, how things change. I remember borrowing diamonds from Boodles for a photo shoot – so precious that they came with a security detail for the day. That was just a standard Monday morning.

A mere blip on the radar, I tell myself, not letting nostalgia get the better of me. My styling days might be over, but nature abhors a vacuum. The sooner I get my medication sorted, the sooner I can explore my options. For now, it's back to my usual prescription. Those new tablets just aren't feasible, sadly. If I reduce the amount I take each day, my symptoms return. When I try a lower dosage instead (hence the pill cutter), it just doesn't deliver. It could be that time is needed to tolerate the drug better or that I am just particularly sensitive to it. Either way, I don't have the bandwidth to find out. *The Tommy Tiernan Show* and ieStyle Live are around the corner, and I need to give my body and mind space to recalibrate before trying a new regime. I might have lost this round, but it's still game on. I'm even warming up to the idea of boxing, which is said to help fight off Parkinson's symptoms. Lord knows I could use a punching bag right now – or a hug. I could use a hug.

* * *

I have one job: to choose a dress, not 40 different looks from different retailers like I used to do. It's a simple brief, yet this level of overthinking suggests I'm trying to figure out string theory. After much trying and not buying, I take Patricia's advice and pull a full-length vintage frock and a pair of Dries Van Noten heels from my wardrobe. Gathering dust, they're only dying for a night out, and so am I.

Tonight, over 300 guests will congregate at Cork's City Hall to join the *Irish Examiner* for the fourth annual instalment of ieStyle Live – the paper's flagship lifestyle event. Showcasing an expert edit of seasonal looks and a special fireside chat with author and comedian Maeve Higgins, the buzz is undeniable.

It's a night of firsts: the first in-person gathering since 2019 and my first year as a guest, not the stylist. To be honest, I'm looking forward to it. Plus, I have the lovely job of selecting winners of the best-dressed award at the end of the night. It's also my first time socialising on this scale with Parkinson's as my plus one. For the first time in a long time, I feel ready.

Behind the Doric columns that flank the entrance to City Hall is a banquet room of familiar faces. Hugs, laughs and long overdue chats punctuate the evening's course of events. It feels great to be dressed up, asking people what they're wearing and what inspires their aesthetic. After years of bland joggers and shapeless knits, everyone dials up the drama. It's a positive sign of the times.

Vickie, my editor, takes me backstage to say hello to everyone, including this year's stylist, with whom I share my best wishes for tonight.

"That was you back when it all started," says Vickie.

"I must confess I'm happy to be on the other side of the runway this time."

"I can only imagine. It's a lot of work."

It certainly is. My mind serves up memories of organising models, pulling and returning clothes and ensuring nothing gets damaged or lost. As a stylist, if something goes wrong, you shoulder the responsibility. There is no room for error, and in the case of live shows, there is one chance to get it right. Nothing feels quite like that dopamine hit when you pull it off, though. Still, it's a measured life for me now. No extremes. No pressure. Neither too much nor too little of anything. The crazy stories I have about dressing celebrities, me modelling on the roof of Bono's hotel after the Beast from the East, the pressure of waiting on a delayed courier to deliver a front cover look with 20 minutes left to shoot – these are artefacts of an earlier me. Out with the old, in with the new, whatever that may be.

While dessert is being served, I excuse myself to go backstage. Before announcing the best-dressed winners, Vickie asks if I would feel comfortable staying on stage to discuss my Parkinson's journey with hosts Brendan Courtney and Sonya Lennon. I feel honoured to do so and can sense my tremor gearing up in anticipation. After presenting the goody bags to our winners, Brendan asks me about life since publicly sharing my diagnosis. There is a static silence across the ballroom as I discuss the incredible support from my *Irish Examiner* article and the current strides in research, especially from University College Cork and the Michael J. Fox Foundation.

"There is hope for a cure, maybe not in my lifetime, but that's why it's so important to me to pay it forward and do what I can to raise awareness, especially of early-onset PD in women." Trying to keep the microphone steady, my body has other plans as it dances between jarring and wavelike motions. There's no hiding it. This is my best version of best; frankly,

I'm OK with that. It is what it is. "I'm a tough old broad," I declare, to which there is a peal of applause.

Uplifted by audience appreciation, I feel a mixture of gratitude and relief, like I'm sharing my story for the first time. A lump forms in my throat when the realisation hits me: people don't see me for my job title or my diagnosis, people see me for me – shaky and all. There is no reason to hide. One foot in front of the other.

As the show wraps and backstage banter subsides, Ciara, one of my editorial colleagues, offers me a lift home. While she grabs her coat from the cloakroom, I wait in the foyer, loosening my swollen feet from their cages of misery. Rookie mistake. One by one, my toes expand, refusing to be sequestered. No amount of wiggling works, so I inhale sharply and jam them back in my shoes. Five hours in four-inch heels after two years in slippers and sneakers – the pain smarts. So does the thought of ice packs and ibuprofen for the next few days. Ping. It's Ciara: she's wrapping something up backstage and will be another few minutes, so I scroll through my emails and WhatsApp to pass the time.

A message from Andy sits unread in the group chat. When I click on it, life immediately changes. Andy has a very rare form of motor neurone disease. I can't believe what I'm reading. His neurologist is hopeful that it is restricted to his leg and will progress slowly. Some patients, Andy says, live for 15 years. I am dumbstruck. MND is a devastating neurological illness. It's like Parkinson's on speed. He might get five years at best; most people get two or three. I am in shock. I read the text again, as if doing so will change the outcome. Nothing changes. Andy is dying.

* * *

The next few days are marred by feelings of futility and confusion. Andy is only in his forties; he is fit and healthy. Maybe it's a misdiagnosis. How can this be happening to him? To feel useful, I start researching house lifts for wheelchairs, hanging on to the promise of another 15 years despite knowing better. *Any one of us could die before Andy does*, I tell myself, convinced chaos theory might somehow spare him. But again, I know better.

His body is turning into a prison. Soon, muscular indiscretions will erase his independence and vital functions. It is not a question of *if* but *when*. I feel immensely guilty for having Parkinson's, like getting off with parole while he receives a death sentence.

To think less than a year ago, Andy was spending the weekend at mine, treating me to dinner, advising me on practical matters, roasting me on things trivial and encouraging me at my highest and lowest. It's not right. None of this is right.

Later that day, while chatting to Julie about tube elevators, home installation and dual rail technology, I receive an email from *The Tommy Tiernan Show* booker confirming my guest appearance next month. I am elated. The opportunity to share my Parkinson's journey on a national platform is a big step in raising awareness about Parkinson's and how it is perceived. Still, a part of me feels conflicted. How can I speak about my life when Andy's future bears so little hope? I keep things quiet. No group text, not a word . . . until, of course, he asks me about the show. He knows I'm waiting to hear back from the booker. Of all people, he is thrilled for me when I share the news, which makes this moment bittersweet. His generosity of spirit in the face of such injustice is a gesture of true friendship. May my heart open as wide as yours, my friend.

November 2022

Sitting in my dressing room, I spot a basket of complementary chocolates and biscuits, which are backlit by halogen bulbs. *Twirl bars! My kind of rider.* I siphon out the ones I like and squirrel them away in my clutch bag for an after-show snack. I don't want a wad of caramel stuck in my tooth now, but I also don't want any to go to waste. Honestly, you can't take me anywhere. A producer for *The Tommy Tiernan Show* knocks on my door and asks to mic me up.

I'm tonight's first guest – no pressure, then. Despite the baby butterflies and my tremor being, well, my tremor, I feel ready.

Margaret, Catherine and Neil are my guests. They're gabbing in the green room over a glass of wine, no doubt. I make a mental note not to look at the front row of the audience, where they'll be sitting. Back in my college Dramsoc days, I would always see Margaret's head of curls a good noggin above the general audience. While performing in *Death and the Maiden*, I could hear sobbing during one of my monologues. I knew it was her. To be clear, I am a distinctly amateur actor. One might argue below average, yet she sniffed and snotted as if I were Meryl Streep in *Sophie's Choice*. Her support is peerless but also mildly distracting. No eye contact with the audience, then.

The runner takes me backstage and cues me to walk out when the compère announces my name. I'm more than sure that Tommy won't know me. With no burden of expectation, all I can do is relax – and I do, smiling through the initial flicker of nerves as I tell him who I am. Like a stage mom, my tremor senses the limelight, encouraging my foot, hand and arm to entertain the crowd. I assure Tommy that I am neither nervous, hungover, nor possessed by a malevolent entity – three things we agree are all possible.

This hyperkinetic start segues into a great talking point: how I now move through life. Much like my chat with Brendan O'Connor, I discuss the prelude to my diagnosis, the 40-plus symptoms of Parkinson's and the impact it has on my body and mind. Astutely, Tommy spots the undulating motion of my tremor, flush with activity before calming and starting again. "That must be exhausting," he observes. I agree, admitting that I'm tired all the time, but also tired of being tired.

I am surprised at my openness. Our conversation feels more personal, as if I'm disclosing my heart to a therapist. Even the pockets of silence between questions feel intimate.

We discuss relationships – familial and romantic. I share my concerns about not being enough for someone or, worse, being too much. "No one wants to be with the sick girl," is what I want to say, paraphrasing Anne Hathaway's character in the Parkinson's rom-com drama *Love & Other Drugs*. Afraid I'll say too much, I settle on an open-ended, albeit rhetorical, understudy, "What's love got to do with it?"

"Do you find it humiliating?" he asks of my condition. Raw and unfiltered, I appreciate his directness and the trust in our give-and-take.

"No," I assert. "I come from a long lineage of stubborn West of Ireland women, and I'll have none of it. I'm not a victim. I've never seen myself as an advocate, but the personal is political and I don't want people to feel that they have to hide. Why should they have to hide? Besides, I make a great cocktail!"

It's true, I do. The unexpected laughter at such a revealing juncture breaks the tension. That's how I like to live my life, Parkinson's or not. I'm not denying my feelings; I'm merely choosing to feel something better.

There's a useful tool in spiritualism, I tell him, commonly referred to as the emotional guidance scale. Feelings run from despair at its lowest to joy at its highest, each with a frequency or vibration. In simple terms, the higher the vibration, the better the feeling. Assuming we do most things in life for the feel-good payback, it makes sense to ascend the scale where possible, thus improving our emotional set-point.

"I think Johnny Rotten said it," I recall. "Anger is an energy. You may not have the energy to get to joy, but you can get to anger, which is still better than being in despair. So long as it's not purposeless, you can channel anger towards hope, which can then become contentment and satisfaction – that's where you want to live."

"It sounds like a fierce amount of work," Tommy admits. He's right. This is my Everest, but this is also my life, and I'll fight for it. Admittedly, I view everything with more intention in the wake of Andy's diagnosis, from how I spend my time to whom I spend it with.

"I have a duty of care to other people in my community, so it's not just about me," I tell him. "You can wind up being very selfish and bitter if you allow it. You can also give it the two fingers up if you want. That's an option."

I'm sure Johnny Rotten would approve. A few seconds of silence hover amicably before Tommy thanks me for coming on the show and we shake hands. It's such a poignant moment, until the part where I walk off stage in the wrong direction. Classic me. And so, laughter prevails – as it should.

* * *

It's the day after Thanksgiving: 3,000 LED cluster lights huddle together like teenagers on a street corner. A star dangles with the energy of a retired pole dancer from what should be the highest bough. This is not my greatest work. Martha Stewart would wince at such delinquency, but has she tried trimming a tree with a tremor? Didn't think so. Nevertheless, I am determined to turn on my lights today. Tradition demands it. Once Santa makes his way to the end of Fifth Avenue and closes the Macy's Thanksgiving Day Parade, it's perfectly acceptable to short-circuit the National Grid in the name of Christmas. With that in mind, I've got two multi-socket extension leads ready to rock.

I'm not usually this dogmatic, but the first anniversary of my Parkinson's diagnosis is only a few weeks away and I insist on maintaining the festive status quo. Every year, I make Nigella Lawson's rocky road bars and a laundry list of sticky baked goodies for family and friends. This year is no different. By day, the kitchen is like a diabetic's warzone. By night, it is a paradigm of organisation: from the disturbingly neat Tupperware drawer to my now alphabetised spice rack. Insomnia, it appears, has its perks. That said, there's only so much tidying and decorating to do and so many boxes of cookies to make. It doesn't matter how busy you are or try to be; sooner or later, you always catch up with yourself. And so, here I am, sitting at the kitchen table, reflecting rather than deflecting as I write a follow-up piece for the *Irish Examiner*: my Parkinson's diagnosis – one year on.

A year later, nothing is new yet virtually everything has changed. My medication is still being tweaked. I have trouble controlling my tremor. My legs are continuously restless. I spend most days in a sleep deficit from the previous night's impromptu dance party.

It's a struggle. Parkinson's disease does not have a return policy (more like a lifetime guarantee), but I won't allow it to call the shots. Every day, I try to understand how to live well with a squatter that claims adverse possession over my body and mind. For the most part, it involves pressing pause until I learn how to move forward. *But for how long?* I wonder.

Life might not happen on my timeline, but the privilege of having a life to live more than makes up for it. Yes, it's frustrating to put my body through a new course of medication. Yes, decision fatigue takes its toll. Yes, it costs time trialling a new treatment, but it's time well spent if my quality of life improves. In the meantime, the future remains conditional, governed by 'if' and populated by possibilities. I know I'll never return to my old way of life, but if there's a chance that I'll feel like my old self again – I'll take it. I'm open to a Christmas miracle. If not now, then when?

* * *

"This could be it, Jules," I grin, scooping melted Brie from the crockpot onto a broken cracker. The tree lights twinkle in agreement.

"I really hope so. It's been a long road for you."

"Twelve months." I raise my glass in mock celebration, chasing the cheese with a mouthful of school-night fizz. Then I remember.

"My appointment at the infusion unit in CUH is January 6th. Will you be my chaperone?"

"Chaperone?"

"The letter from the hospital says I need a family member or a main caregiver to accompany me on the day." I roll my eyes in apology, grabbing the envelope with the plastic window from the top of the coffee maker.

"Of course I will." Without hesitation, she puts the details into her phone.

I fidget in my seat. *God, I hate asking.* "This chronic illness malarkey isn't exactly set up for single people. If you ever move, I'll have to hire someone as my hospital escort. Surely there's an app for that."

Julie shakes her head in comic disapproval. "Oh, Annie. That sounds like the plot of a dodgy film pitch."

"I used to think a bachelor with moderate baggage and decent dinner reservations was sexy. Now, someone I can carpool with for routine medical procedures has a ring to it. I'm probably better off cruising the middle aisle at Aldi. You can tell a lot by a person's Specialbuys taste."

Julie changes the subject to more practical matters. "Tell me more about this injection."

"Well, I began taking an ancillary oral drug in mid-November after *The Tommy Tiernan Show*. It's said to reduce resting tremors by 70 per cent. So far, nothing."

"Not again." Julie's expression flattens. False starts and false hopes go hand in hand.

"That's why I've decided to go the injection route," I assure her. "As awkward as it seems to administer a needle a few times a day, it's no different than a diabetic with insulin. The dopamine is delivered beneath the skin rather than through the gut. This means I can get relief in seven minutes as opposed to waiting the best part of an hour with a tablet, which is crucial, especially when I wake up in pain at night."

Julie exhales. "That in itself is worth it."

"There's just one thing," I add, having learned the art of the shit sandwich from my sister, Margaret. "It's a dopamine agonist, which I've been panicky about, but the fact that it's liquid means the drug doesn't stay in my system long enough for it to negatively impact the reward centre of the brain."

"I'd imagine that would minimise the risk of developing an impulse control disorder."

"Exactly!" I beam. "Our new Parkinson's nurse, who started at CUH in September, has been such a great help. I have a few more tests at my GP before Christmas. Then, I'm good to go. If this works, it could be a legitimate Christmas miracle: the 'move over in the crib, baby Jesus' kind. If not, I guess I'll have to give the dopamine agonist tablets a try." Not knowing what comes next, I shrug. It feels appropriate.

As we sit in uncertainty, I pour another round of school-night fizz. Julie raises a toast. "Here's to good health and good luck. May you get a decent dose of both."

"Cheers!" We clink glasses and continue chatting about the kids' presents, plans for Christmas dinner and how we both think the Elf on the Shelf is a bit creepy. It's a relief to talk about Santa and the usual festive activities. I take this as a sign of good things to come: a thrill of hope wrapped in the mundane. This could be it.

January 2023

Today, I'm learning how to inject myself. I'm still not a fan of needles, despite my foray with acupuncture, but I'm willing to give anything a go. Julie drives me to the hospital, where I meet with the CUH Parkinson's nurse and the apomorphine nurse, who will show me how to use the apomorphine pen – a subcutaneous dopamine delivery system that can provide relief from tremors up to ten times a day. Contrary to what the name suggests, apomorphine is not morphine. It is neither an analgesic nor an opioid. It is, however, famously feted by Beat Generation writer William S. Burroughs in his book *Naked Lunch* as an antidote to his long-term drug addiction.

This trivia is neither here nor there, nor are my dopamine levels. We're all stuck in the middle somewhere in life.

As a medication lightweight, I've been prescribed anti-nausea tablets to prepare for today's appointment. There is a strong possibility I might feel sick as they scale the treatment to assess my optimal dose. Considering I look away whenever my GP takes blood, I am surprised at how confidently I pinch and pierce my belly fat with liquid dopamine. I can take one milligram out of a potential ten so far without feeling sick. This is a promising start. By my second milligram, I feel woozy and my resting heart rate drops considerably. What's more, my eyes won't stay open. I assume the foetal position on the PVC examination chair while one of the nurses brings me a cup of tea and a biscuit. So nauseated I can barely move, this might be the worst hangover I never had. Ten minutes later, the bargaining with God passes and disappointment fills the void.

To no one's surprise, I'm not a successful candidate for treatment due to my body's reaction at such a low dosage. I can't help but feel defeated. After 13 months and various combinations of drugs, the prospect of being able to administer medication when I need it, to be in control of my body again, is now lost. The CUH Parkinson's nurse reassures me there are other possibilities, including a patch that has come on the market, which might prove more user-friendly. Dr Sweeney and I discuss these options over email, giving me time to do some research before our next appointment in February.

I worry about how I'll fare at reduced capacity over the next four weeks: the anxiety of meeting deadlines, the financial insecurity, wondering if the next drug will be 'the one'. It's getting tiresome. When Julie drops me home, I change into my pyjamas and pass out cold for three hours on the sofa.

The next few days are trying. My hands are almost useless between the incessant tremor and the rigidity that leaves my fingers stiff and unable to bend. My legs and feet aren't much better. I get this dull, intense ache in the front of my thighs about an hour or two before I go to bed. Hot water bottles help ease the soreness so that I can sleep, yet that familiar jerking pain still wakes me up at silly o'clock in the morning when my dopamine is at its lowest. The half tablet I usually take in emergencies doesn't seem to have the same effect, but I'm afraid to take a full one without first speaking to Dr Sweeney. The more L-dopa in the system, the more dyskinesia is likely. Trading off one twitch for another doesn't seem like the best deal.

I don't even have the strength to fight it, physical or otherwise. I think back to last weekend when Patricia and I were looking at fabric in the Woolen Mills upholstery store. I struggled to hold the bolt of material upright for her while she answered her phone. Some days still feel like a battle. I just don't know what to do.

Getting the balance right takes time, or so I tell myself. Trust the process. Exhaust all options. Throw everything at it. Throwing everything at it, however, *is* exhausting. It's dull, repetitive and requires a lot of energy, especially for one person.

Waiting is the hard part. Waiting for the pain to ease and the dopamine to kick in, waiting for the shaking to subside, waiting to fall back to sleep when my body insists on moving. Waiting to feel like myself again.

With my patience continuously tested, everyday tasks and habits become little pockets of resistance – mental and physical minefields that need to be traversed. My body is always pulsing, contracting and wilfully kinetic, even at rest. My mind is still sharp but often in need of a break.

But there is no break, not with Parkinson's. I begin to question my faith in the future, a higher power and me. Do I have the moxie to stay the course? Who am I to assume things will work out in my favour? Sometimes life is chaotic, unpredictable and, certainly, not fair. Often it winds up being completely different to what we expected, whether good or bad. Maybe this is as good as it gets? I thought I could call the shots, but I can't. It's bigger than me – bigger than I realise.

CHAPTER SEVEN

Miracles

Persistence pays

January 2023

It starts with a click. That sinking feeling. Deadbolt. Then a flashback. *No, not again. Not now.* I forgot my keys. I know this because I'm wearing a T-shirt and pyjama bottoms. No pockets. Definitely no keys. In each hand is a bag of rubbish. No phone either. My tremor kicks in. Logic dips out. I call the elevator and take three floors' worth of deep breaths to the mezzanine. *Let me at least put this rubbish away*, I think, before remembering the communal shed is locked. How could I forget my keys – *again*?

Julie has a spare set. She's smart like that. Smarter than me, who has had to call on her good graces twice in the past six months. Three times and the universe automatically mandates a lesson learned the hard way. The celestial scorekeeper scorns my complacency, brain fog and childlike inability to remember the simplest things. So she makes this an *oopsie* I'll never forget.

It's late. Eight p.m. late. According to the weather forecast, it's also the coldest day of the year. Here I am in furry slippers with two bags of rubbish, no keys and no phone as I begin the 15-minute uphill walk to Julie's house in the dark.

Grateful for small mercies, I console myself that no one can see me in the low glare of dipped headlights. Then it starts to hail. Or is that snow? Icy pellets hit my face with contempt. I can feel the skin of my big toe chafing against wet fleece with each step. *Not far to go*, I tell myself, all the while wondering how long it takes for hypothermia to set in.

I arrive at Julie's house. My hands are numb, so numb I can't ring the doorbell. Instead, I bang on a pane of opaque glass with my right elbow, which is currently the only body part I can feel. The door opens.

"Hi, is your mom home?"

Her daughter smiles politely. My harried expression speaks volumes. She's met me before, but not like this – a wet, limping iteration of my usual self.

"Annie, come on in." A familiar voice approaches from the hallway. Julie's husband assumes door duty and ushers me indoors.

"I forgot my keys," I mumble.

"Ah, you poor thing. You're freezing. Here, I'll take those for you," he says, reaching for the bags.

I retract. "It's OK, really," I implore. "I'll bring them home with me." Either I have a survivalist attachment to the recycling (a new low), or I am subconsciously refusing to have others deal with my garbage – probably the latter. The kitchen door opens. I hear Julie's maternal voice. Tea is being made. A sweater is being offered. Distracted, I release the hostages to Julie's husband, who repatriates them into their green bin.

"I'm so sorry. I forgot my keys. I forgot my phone. I had to walk in the snow. I was carrying rubbish ..." Julie actively listens as I deliver the world's worst TED Talk from the middle of the kitchen floor in wet slippers and a pool of self-pity.

Soothing words follow. I feel like a burden. Julie drives me home and ensures I am locked *inside* my apartment. I spot my keys on the kitchen counter and remember I have a pompom in the odds and sods drawer. Unspeakably large, it can double as a keyring and an agent of shame. Having a lot on my mind is no excuse – not anymore. So, the injection route didn't work out. So, it's back to the drawing board. So what? Try again. And again. And again, if needs be. A door is bound to open.

* * *

"Hello?" I answer the phone, dreaming it's the front door.
"I'm so sorry. Did I wake you?"
"What time is it?" I ask, not even sure who's calling.
"It's a little after 11 a.m. I rang you a few times this morning, but you didn't pick up."
The Dublin accent is familiar. It's Andy. I bolt upright, now fully awake. "Is everything OK?" I blurt. Andy is coming to Cork this weekend to catch up with a group of our friends in Cobh. I told him to stay at my place as it's better suited to his wheelchair, but he wanted to stay in Cobh for convenience.
"Don't panic. There's been a change of plans. I'm on the train to Cork and just wanted to check if it's OK that I stay with you. Olly and Alan are collecting me from Kent Station at 1.45 p.m., so I should be at your apartment around the two-ish mark."
"Of course!" It's more than OK. I'm delighted, albeit mildly flustered. My Tesco delivery doesn't arrive until tomorrow so the cupboards are bare bar a few cans of beans, chicken stock and condiments of some description. I hate being unprepared. Winging it gives me anxiety. *Can I shower, clean the apartment and make lunch for four people in less than three hours?* I ask myself as I check the refrigerator and realise I'm also out of milk and coffee. I guess I'm running to the shops too.

Ping.
We're outside.

Half-panting, I put my damp hair into a makeshift bun as I make my way to the living room window. I wave to Olly, who is getting the bags from the boot. Alan holds the passenger door for Andy, who hoists himself into his wheelchair. The elevator is small, so I buzz them up to my apartment as I quickly set the kitchen table. A faint chime from the hallway pre-empts their arrival. I open the door to big smiles, hugs and belated New Year wishes.

"Is that homemade soup I smell?" asks Olly. I show them inside, telling Alan to make a wish on his first visit to the apartment. This time last year, Andy was carrying the bags and getting settled into the Eames chair. Today, I push it aside to make room for his new wheeled quarters. Things look different but feel the same.

We have a Tuscan beef stew and some crusty bread for lunch and catch up on all sorts of everything before Alan leaves to go back to work. The rest of us continue putting the world to rights for several hours. We order an Indian takeaway that evening as Ru Paul entertains us with another drag race over dinner. It's late. Olly has to get home but arranges to bring us to Cobh tomorrow, where we're meeting the others for lunch – a mini-reunion.

Andy and I stay up chatting a while longer. He tries to manoeuvre himself onto the sofa from his chair. It's a struggle: his arms are weak, yet needed to move his immobile trunk. It's difficult to watch. "I know you know this," I say, "but shout if you want me to help. The last thing you need is me in your way if you can manage on your own."

"I will. Thanks, Ams." Honesty dissolves the tension, leaving ease in its wake. The following afternoon, a gaggle of us decamp to the Titanic Bar and Grill – what was once the ticketing office for the White Star Line. Grandma would have boarded the RMS *Samaria* to the USA with her brother not so far from here. I wonder if they were scared. It breaks my heart to think that the next time she returned to Ireland, 70 years later, would be her first and last trip home.

Why is life so tough for some people? I look at everyone embracing Andy, some crying, others waiting until later. What a crushing coincidence that this visit to Cobh might well be his last, too.

After hours of chats, food and good company, Andy and I head back to my place to watch my appearance on *The Tommy Tiernan Show*. The cab driver asks us about our night. Andy tells him we met up with friends he's known for years and that he is dying. Silence. The driver extends his sympathy as Andy chats to him about MND. I am stunned. Hearing Andy say those words makes it real, like he's preparing himself for what's ahead.

Back in the apartment, we sit side by side on the sofa as the opening credits roll at 9.30 p.m. I'm nervous. Nervous about how I'll appear on TV. Nervous about sharing this moment with Andy, who, only an hour earlier, admitted he is dying. Words such as 'progressing' are no longer adequate to describe his condition. Now, he doesn't sugarcoat it. He doesn't have time.

Reliving my experience on TV, I realise how lucky I am and what a privilege it is to share my story. I'm still able to talk, walk, breathe and swallow – small miracles often taken for granted. Getting ready to go to bed, Andy calls me into his room and asks if I can help him get from the chair onto the mattress. We chit-chat about tomorrow's plans: lunch at Fifi's house in Cobh before he heads to Clonakilty on a break with the boys. I remind him there's a fresh batch of rocky road on the kitchen table and to help himself. Things look different, but now they *feel* different. I kiss him on the forehead and say goodnight. These will be some of our last moments together.

February 2023

I remember cycling to Lady's Well in Athenry with my friends as an early teen. It was the mid-80s, the peak era of moving statues. We were fascinated by the phenomenon and determined to have an experience to share with the world. Standing before the grotto, we stared at Our Lady, silently repeating her prayer, hoping to spot a tear, as was reported in other towns. The most we got was eye strain. Now and again, we made the two-kilometre pilgrimage on our bikes, optimistic that a miracle awaited. Miracles, of course, were everywhere: quiet ones that didn't make the nine o'clock news. We didn't see them. We were looking for the sparkle. This I understood later in life, as I sought out the divine, unaware of its presence all along.

* * *

I'm collecting my new medication from the pharmacy today. Dr Sweeney supported my request to start on a dopamine agonist in the form of a transdermal patch. As the delivery system bypasses the gut, it might improve absorption, given my persistent issues in that department. The online forums seem to back its efficacy, with many people hailing it as a wonder drug, especially for restless legs and tremors. The main drawbacks are nausea in the first few days and a reduced appetite, with some users on Reddit reporting having lost up to two stone. My care team strongly advises me to read the prescription literature, especially about impulse control disorders. Having such an open and honest rapport with my consultant and Parkinson's nurse, I feel confident in sharing any potential behavioural changes, should they occur.

I opt to embark on the new course of medication tomorrow morning. It's scalable: a two milligram transdermal patch taken daily for one week increased to four milligrams from then on. I have a Parkinson's charity fundraising meeting in Cork Coffee Roasters at 10 a.m., but I should be home by midday, in case I start to feel unwell.

As predicted, I am home bang on noon – so far, so good, bar some fatigue. A nap sounds like a good idea. Barely a wrinkle in the duvet, I wake after two and a half hours and attempt to get out of bed, which fails miserably. Everything is spinning. This must be what it feels like in one of those zero-gravity rooms. I want to be sick, but I can't. The only respite I get is by lying prone. These hampered efforts continue until 7.30 p.m. when I make it to the kitchen for a cup of tea. I don't have any anti-nausea tablets left from last month's injection trial, but I do have ones for motion sickness, which I typically reserve for the journey to Inishbofin. Who knows? It might stop the vertigo.

The CUH Parkinson's nurse calls me the next day to see how I'm getting on. I tell her about the queasiness, which comes in waves and shows no signs of abating. She advises me to take domperidone as opposed to the motion sickness tablets, which, in the long-term, can mimic the symptoms of Parkinson's and make it seem worse. I call my GP to request a prescription and ask Julie to collect it after work if she has time. She comes bearing a first aid kit of medication, Lucozade, chicken noodle soup and ice cream. "You look awful, Annie." She tilts her head with a mother's pity. She's not wrong.

"A small trade-off," I admit, sharing my delight at having slept last night and the noticeable reduction in my restless legs and tremors. "Trust issues with medication aside, the patch looks promising."

Julie pops two tablets from the blister pack for me, which I swig with orange fizz. "I'd say they're sick of seeing me at the pharmacy. This is my millionth script already."

I pause.

Julie picks up on my hesitation. "What's up?" she asks, taking a seat beside me on the bed.

"It's nothing—"

"—which means it's something, Annie."

"I'm annoyed at myself, that's all. Had I gone the dopamine agonist route earlier, I could have spared myself months of grief. I just wish I hadn't been so risk-averse."

"Shoulda, woulda, coulda. You did the right thing to take things slow and scale up. This medication that you're on could have just as easily not worked. No one knows. Everything is a risk to some degree. I also remember you telling me that the chance of compulsive behaviour can happen at any stage in your treatment. Then again it may not. It's a risk, nonetheless. You need to trust your judgement more."

She's right. I'm still caught in the tailwinds of my decision to move to Dublin. I need to move on.

"Julie ... I also want to say thanks. I feel like I've been leaning on you a lot recently, what with the keys the other night—"

"And the rubbish. Don't forget the rubbish." Julie does her best to suppress a cheeky grin.

"*And* the rubbish." I hide my face in my hands, mortified. Giggles follow.

"What good is a friend, Annie, if they can't do your recycling?"

"Or your *punding*, for that matter." Julie looks puzzled so I consult Google on my phone. "Listen to this: punding is the compulsive need to carry out repetitive motor behaviour such as sorting materials you are no longer using, counting small objects, lining them up and counting them again, or taking everything out of the drawer, examining it and doing it all over again."

"What does this have to do with rubbish?" Julie asks.

"If I do draw the short straw with the dopamine agonists, I think punding is a good bet as potential ICDs go." I brandish the patch information leaflet – my bedside reading. "It's just a shame I'm no longer decluttering people's wardrobes. It could be a lucrative number, provided I could be stopped before undoing all my good work. I could, of course, pivot into stocktaking as Neil suggests," I kid.

"Or you could pund away at my place. I'll be up to my neck in boxes before we move next month," she groans. "The thought of starting over again in a new house is daunting – packing and unpacking just to live three kilometres away!" She slumps in objection.

"All joking aside, be sure to recruit me. You know tidying and organising is my not-so-secret hobby."

Julie stifles a prescient yawn. "We'll all keep an eye out for you," she says, gathering her tote bag and scarf, "but I'm sure you can safely park punding for the moment. How about you enjoy sleeping through the night again, being able to type, no restless legs? It's a blessed relief." She smiles, tilting her head once more in motherly mode. "Worry less, live more. You deserve it."

March 2023

It's International Women's Day. I am part of a panel of three speakers invited by the *Irish Examiner* to discuss this year's theme: embracing equity. I am still reeling from the surprise of being voted by our readers as one of the 100 Women Changing Ireland – a celebration of those making positive waves across the country. It's a far cry from where I was last year: getting to grips with my medication and soft-launching my diagnosis to strangers. I feel lucky that I get to share my lived experience of Parkinson's and can encourage others to do the same. Personal advocacy is more than storytelling; it's a powerful instrument of change. Speaking of which, I'll be heading home to pack after we wrap. Neil and I are flying to Sicily tomorrow for a mini break. We both need vitamin D and time out from the day to day. With my health turning a corner and me turning 50 in two months, now feels like the best time to follow the sun.

Arriving the following evening in Palermo, we head out for a dinner of squid ink pasta and salted cod at a local trattoria. Forgetting that primo and secondo courses leave little room for dessert, we opt for a walk through the cobblestone streets punctuated by shrines to Santa Rosalia, who is said to have eradicated Palermo's 1624 plague. Although it's a little after ten, the nighttime temperature still reads as light-blazer-appropriate, a far cry from the previous night's sudden snowfall at home.

We stop for an Aperol Spritz just off Piazza Bellini. Sitting outside on indoor furniture underneath rows of fairy lights, I see a plaque with a quote from Nelson Mandela hanging overhead: "A winner is just a dreamer who never gave up." We finish our nightcaps and walk past the adjacent honesty library decorated with a replica of Banksy's *Flower Thrower.* As we near the Arab–Norman square, we hear classical music. A group of students enact a Regency flash mob in front of Santa Caterina church, dancing quadrilles under the light of a new moon. Neil and I are in awe, like kids seeing something for the first time.

Briefly forgetting our ages, we take a quick selfie with the naked statues at the Fontana Pretoria (known colloquially as the Fountain of Shame) before returning to the hotel. That photo captures pure joy. Our big giddy grins and the inky residue on my teeth give it away.

* * *

Three days and three nights don't technically qualify as a vacation, but the break works wonders in recharging my batteries. Next month, I have several events for Parkinson's Awareness Week scheduled, including the launch of my Parkinson's podcast with the *Irish Examiner* and a guest speaker spot at the Parkinson's Ireland National Conference. Plus, I have a front cover photo for my fiftieth birthday feature in *Weekend* magazine and a press call for the fundraising event I'm hosting – both on the same day. My dance card is filling up, and I'm conscious that I might not see Mom until summer. So, we arrange for her to come to Cork at the end of the month for lunching, shopping and catching up – in no particular order.

"You've lost a lot of weight, dear," Mom says from the kitchen as I wheel her suitcase into the guest room. She's forthright but fair, a gene she inherited from Nana.

"I know," I confess from a distance. "The patch is working wonders, but my appetite isn't what it used to be. At least I don't have that awful nausea anymore." Changing the subject,

I tell Mom to close her eyes as I walk towards her with my hands behind my back. "I have a surprise for you."

"You know, dear, I love what you did with those mirrors. These must be new. The last time I was here—"

"Mom, pay attention." I chuckle while placing a decorative maiolica tile in the palms of her hands.

"Sorry, it's not properly wrapped."

"Oh, dear. You shouldn't have spent your money on me," she coos, removing the protective bubble sheet. Her fingers dance over the yellow and blue hand-painted flourishes. "It's simply beautiful."

"A small token," I admit, blaming budget airline restrictions, "but it's meant to bring good luck."

We hug and then sit down for a good natter, mainly about my trip to Palermo and a book Mom read recently about the Moorish influence on Italian ceramics. An ardent history buff, her topic of choice is the Roman Empire, followed by Ancient Egypt and almost any Italian-adjacent matter a close third. Her factual knowledge is first class. Mine is sketchy at best, with dates distilled to eras and historic figures referred to as "yer man" or "King What's His Name".

Ping. Prompted by the calendar alarm on my phone, our lunch reservation at Barry's is in 20 minutes. "I better call a cab," I remark, grabbing our coats and bags while the app waits to see which drivers are free.

Arriving just before the lunch crowd, we get a window seat with lovely midday light. As the server brings over the menus, Mom searches for her glasses. "I'll save you time, Mom. You've got to try their Reuben. It's amazing."

When it comes to food, I don't dilly-dally, especially being the family's youngest. If you want to see natural selection in action, put a hot pizza in front of five hungry kids. So, yes,

I'm the person who consults the online menu before making a reservation and skips starters to get to the main course. Both peckish for a piece of New York nostalgia, we place the same order. I smile at Mom, happy to be spending this time together, and I yelp with delight when two plates of Swiss cheese and spiced beef with sauerkraut on rye make their way to our table. After a few bites, I feel full – Christmas dinner full. Despite feeling hungry earlier, I physically can't eat anymore.

"Are you OK?" Mom signals to the half sandwich on my plate, left untouched. I sigh, rubbing my belly. "I wish I could finish it. I don't know why my body is reacting like this. I mean, I ate all around me in Palermo."

"It might be the medication. Your appetite can change for a variety of reasons," she observes, taking a sip of her coffee.

"Now, dear. It may well settle, but if it continues, please speak to your doctor about it, in case there are any underlying issues." When Mom begins a sentence with "now dear" (not to be confused with a singular "dear"), it means one of two things: she's either telling you something you need to hear (so listen up) or she's giving you a polite albeit public dressing-down. Mine, thankfully, is the former.

"I don't need to tell you this." Mom waves her hand as if dismissing the obvious. "You're a grown woman, but I *am* your mother and that will never change." She folds her arms with a loving smirk, happy to have said her peace.

"It's more a cause for disappointment rather than concern," I reassure her. "I do love my food, but I'll keep an eye on it."

After lunch, we have plans for retail therapy – some summer tops, maybe new sheets and pillowcases – before relaxing at home with a Rick Stein travel documentary, Mom's favourite.

The following morning, I'm not very hungry. "That won't keep you full, dear." She points to two peanut butter oatcakes on my plate, tapping her finger in gentle Morse code judgement. It does keep me full. That's the issue. Usually, I have something more substantial, plus a second breakfast after two hours. Then I plan what to have for dinner before I even have lunch. The convivial (albeit insistent) food chatter that occupies my head is now quieter, for the most part. I'm grateful for Mom's frank observations over the past two days. Living alone can sometimes feel like an echo chamber, insulated from the viewpoints of others. I always prefer to hear what I need rather than be told what I want, but, truthfully, I'd rather have an iffy appetite than give up this patch. I can't have another miracle slip through my fingers. Habituation is a pain in the arse but, as Mom always says, "This too shall pass". Let's hope so.

* * *

I'm working again. Working slowly but with barely a tremor. Working without my legs jerking in pain. To be able to sit still at my desk without my body and mind constantly activated means I can focus and get things done. For me, it feels like a stay of execution from the time I spend ruminating whether my latest twitch is a precursor to God knows what. And so, I'm making up for lost time, at my new pace.

Experts say I'm supposed to make like Goldilocks: not too little, not too much. Admittedly, I have yet to find that middle ground. When the realities of life hit, such as rent and bills, going with the flow can seem a privileged pursuit. To say I'm working on it would be a lie, as I'm probably actually working on my next article or the new podcast.

Don't get me wrong. I'm full of appreciation for my current health and I do everything I can to maintain it, which is work in itself. That said, I can also appreciate that I can, sustain a semblance of a career. This is also a privilege. And so, for now, I work.

* * *

After Mom leaves, I start recording a promo for my new podcast in the guest bedroom, which doubles as a home studio. By that, I mean I can do a few clean takes on my phone app without interruptions from passing traffic, which wouldn't be possible at my kitchen table. Plus, the incriminating number of decorative pillows helps absorb any background noise.

> Join Annmarie O'Connor, *Irish Examiner* columnist and Parkinson's advocate, for *Living Your Best Life*, a special podcast series launching Tuesday, 11th April – World Parkinson's Day. Sharing personal stories from the Irish Parkinson's community, expect an uplifting mix of insight, grit and humour in this insider's guide to living well.

Pre-promotion starts next week, so I send the best take to production to be layered with a music bed. Meanwhile, we've got to record five episodes in two days at the end of this week, which I'm excited about. My objective with this podcast is to dismantle stereotypes and create positive visibility for people with Parkinson's. With the help of Parkinson's Ireland, the guest lineup is designed to shed light on lived experiences – male and female, early- and late-onset, spouses and carers – focusing on how people overcome obstacles and the tools they use to thrive. Being vulnerable enough to share details of our lives will hopefully go some way to alleviate fear for those on a similar journey. I want people to know that there is life with Parkinson's.

Like most things, though, you get back what you put in. For me, the payoff, after months of challenges, is using my platform to support the Parkinson's community. I'm lucky, I'll admit. And, yes, the stubborn West of Ireland genes help.

April 2023

I'm at the *Irish Examiner* office ooh-ing and aah-ing at the slick, new podcast suite. Knowing I'm in good hands with our production manager, Jim, I feel confident, which will, in turn, put our guests at ease. So will the plates of pastries laid out in the boardroom. Life is sweeter with a cinnamon bun and a nice cup of coffee – or so I tell myself before reporting for hosting duties.

Ping. I wipe my icing-clad fingers on a nearby napkin and check my phone. It's a text from Andy in the group chat.

The health service is providing him with extra help: two people to get him up and washed every morning and again in the evening to get him to bed. Every day, a little bit of him slips away. Sympathetic words feel meaningless and hollow. We'll see more messages like this. It's only the beginning.

Ping. It's Jerome, our first podcast guest. He's dropping the kids at school and is caught in traffic. He'll be another ten minutes. Ping. It's Vickie, my boss, checking if I'm OK. She's on her way. I update Jim on Jerome's estimated arrival time and head upstairs to reception to greet him. Once we are all situated and the microphones are on, Jim counts me in: 5-4-3-2-1. As I listen to the incredible stories of people with Parkinson's, I notice a common thread. Regardless of age, gender, onset or symptoms, there is always hope. It's the sparkle I sought as a teen – my quiet miracle. I wish I could say the same for Andy. Sometimes, the lens we call perspective is unduly sharp. We are watching him die as our lives go on. No miracle here. No. Not today.

* * *

I'm standing at the bus shelter, playing the waiting game with other commuters, when two girls walk by. One stops and looks straight at me – mouth open at full aperture – while the other hovers a pace or two ahead. I run the mental numbers. *Do I know this person? How do I know her? A name? Any name. Come on, brain!*

"You're that girl from the podcast!"

Low dopamine leaves me with a blank stare.

"—the Parkinson's podcast."

Thankful for the clarification, I confirm that's me. If only she'd do the same.

"Oh my god, I can't believe this is happening." Her exclamation draws curious looks from the waiting commuters and a disappointed "pfft" from someone hoping for a more interesting sighting.

"I drove up from Ennis this morning to meet my friend for lunch." She turns to the other girl who is now beside her. "This is Caroline and I'm Tanya."

Thank God!

We acknowledge each other with overlapping "nice to meet you" exchanges.

"Anyway," she continues, "I just listened to two episodes in the car and, oh my God, I was in tears."

She puts her hand on her heart.

"—good tears," she is quick to point out.

"You see, my mom has Parkinson's, and I often feel guilty about not being able to connect with her like I used to – as if the PD is standing in the way. But in the two-hour drive to Cork, I already understand her better. My heart feels lighter. It's like this information came to me at just the right time."

She shakes her head in amazement. "I still can't believe I met you like this."

Getting out her phone, she follows me on Instagram, then asks if she can hug me before she and Caroline continue down the main street. Two strangers embracing at a bus stop two minutes after a chance meeting. Is this a coincidence . . . or is it fate?

The bus has yet to arrive, but I need a moment to process this unexpected encounter. Maybe there is no such thing as a happy accident. The idea that we are all connected, that some purpose exists in this often inscrutable life is heartening. I wish I could say the same for the bus, which is testing my patience. And, so, I continue to wait, telling myself that divine timing is playing its part.

* * *

The medication alarm on my phone goes off. Only ten minutes until the train hits Heuston Station. I take my yellow pill with a slug of water, gather my things and stand between the carriage doors, unsure from which I will alight at the platform. No time to waste. On today's agenda is visiting Andy and getting something to wear for next month's charity lunch. My changing body shape means much of what I own doesn't fit me. Plus, I want something fresh to represent a new start. Something bright might be nice. After hours of seeing beige, beige and more beige, I call time on my bright idea and text Andy to see if it's convenient for me to pop over. Divinely timed, I hop in a cab to his place before his home help arrives, which will be in the next hour. That should allow for a quick life debrief and some necessary gossip. Andy texts me to say that the door is unlocked and to let myself in. I press the buzzer out of habit and as a heads-up.

"It's just me!" I shout as I cross the threshold. To the side of the corridor in what used to be the front room is a single bed fitted with a medical mattress to prevent pressure sores.

"I'm in the sitting room, Ams."

I feel a lump in my throat. My inner critic gets wind of it; she's not pleased. *Get it together, Annmarie, and don't you dare think of crying!*

"Fancy new wheels!" I wolf whistle as I spot Andy in his swanky motorised chair, forgetting he's now too weak for a manual one. I kiss him on the forehead before getting comfy on the sofa and talking *way* too much. "No, I won't have tea. I might get the late train home. Maybe I'll stay the night at Margaret's. I'm not sure. Did the builders finish the retrofitting?" Sensing my nerves, he steers the conversation from small talk to what's happening in my life: my new meds, the podcast and next month's fundraiser. Then, beautifully blunt, "You lost weight."

There's my Andy, right on cue. I relax in an instant. "It's the medication," I say. His eyes know more. He's too tired to read me the riot act; I can tell by his sloped shoulders. Instead, he tells me to mind myself and changes the subject to dating.

"Are you seeing anyone at the moment?"

"Me?" I exclaim with a bit too much vigour. "Hardly." Andy has a history of keeping tabs on my inconsistent dating life. "It's all about footfall," he would tell me, insisting I get out more, whatever that looks like, say yes to new things and make myself "visible". He's like Dr Phil if Dr Phil started sentences with, "Let me just stop you there."

I'm waiting for his cue, but he refrains. "Don't leave it too long." That's all he says. I check my phone and realise our time is nearly up. As I put on my coat, he brings up my birthday, determined I do something on May 18th.

"Be sure you mark it." His tone is quietly assertive. "It's important you do." Although I assure him I will, he knows I won't. "Best of luck with the fundraiser. You'll be brilliant, but make sure to enjoy yourself and let us know how you get on." I promise, but not before he posts a selfie of us in the group chat. Just as I'm about to leave, a car pulls up. It's the home help. Couldn't have timed it better.

May 2023

It's my birthday: May 18th. I'm 50 today. Fifty. Imagine. I try not to. Instead, I get ready as I usually do, with no plans to do anything special. The video panel on my wall lights up with a cacophonous buzz. I squint at the monitor to see who it is. It's hard to tell behind what looks like a bouquet.

"Wait, I'm coming down now," I say, pressing the release on the door lock. I emerge from the elevator to an enormous floral arrangement with arms and legs.

"Can you manage, love?" asks a voice behind the sprays of lilies and roses.

I offer a cavalier "No bother" and shuffle back to the lift with my gift. Upstairs in the apartment, I search for a vase big enough to accommodate this statement of intent. That's when I spot a small white card taped inside the stiff folds of cellophane. It's from Andy. He is marking my day for me. I text him immediately to thank him. *You shouldn't have.* Feeling slightly guilty for breaking my promise, I continue with my plans for a day that happens to be my birthday: nothing to report.

* * *

BEEP. BEEP. BEEP.

Later that evening, I'm standing on top of a high, wobbly stool, trying to silence the ceiling fire alarm while not plummeting to my demise.

"I've never been to an escape room. But if I did. I bet you it would sound like this." BEEP. BEEP. BEEP.

"Don't worry, we'll sort it out." Maureen gives me the standard-issue-approved support script from the other end of the phone while I try to establish the chirping source.

"Is it coming from another room?"

"I don't think so," I tell her as I cautiously dismount the stool, distracted by beeps bouncing off the walls. "I checked all the units at least twice. If I don't figure this out, I'll have to wait until I can contact maintenance in the morning. My neighbours are going to hate me!"

"Have you tried the hot press?"

Well, well, well. Above the piles of neatly stacked bath towels are a smoke alarm *and* a carbon monoxide detector. With equal parts relief and rage, I dismantle one and silence the other, unsure which is the offender.

Maureen urges me to get some sleep and wishes me a happy birthday while I open all the apartment windows. Appearing on RIP.ie is not the way I intend to mark the day. So much for having nothing to report. As I change into my pyjamas, I begin to wonder. *Is this a sign from the universe? Does something in my interior world need attention?* The conversation with Andy about my love life comes to mind, which I dismiss as overthinking and turn off the lights.

I email maintenance the following morning. No show. Overtired from the night before, I make a point of going to bed early.

Two hours after I fall asleep: BEEP. BEEP. BEEP.

No, not again. What sorcery is this? I silenced it last night!

Unbeknownst to me, the hush button lasts for 24 hours, after which it beeps again to remind you not to die of carbon monoxide poisoning. I fumble the duvet, find my glasses and check the alarm brand name. I Google it only to discover the chirping reactivates unless a special battery is replaced – the one that I'm guessing maintenance has. With inexpert hands and a fit of pique, I rip off the unit, leave it on the kitchen table and go back to bed. I can't be bothered opening a window. I'm not even tired anymore. Mildly traumatised – but not tired.

Around noon the following day, maintenance arrives.

"Really sorry, there was a bit of a mix-up." A pair of mesmerising azure eyes appear at the door. Something tells me this guy is kept busy replacing perfectly good alarms.

"Come on in," I say. I can feel my pupils dilate into cartoon love hearts.

I show him into the bedroom and start babbling about it being my birthday and the alarm going off and how I disconnected one alarm and pushed the hush button on the other because I didn't want to wake up my neighbours, and then I found out it happens again, you know, because of the special battery, but there's another one in the guest bedroom and I think there's one in the sitting room. I'm not too sure. It could just be the security alarm. It's worth checking, I guess. All these alarms. It's hard to keep up.

Babble. Babble. Babble. It's obvious I don't get out much.

"Yeah, about these batteries: they will chirp like mad unless you change them. They're made that way so that you do something about it. Most people would rather put the thing on silent indefinitely than change them."

"Change is hard," I sigh.

He starts talking about pipes and flues, asking me questions I don't know how to answer, ensuring it's nothing more than a dead battery. "You should be good for about another four years," he nods, seeing himself out, clearly unphased by my amateur flirting skills.

A lot can change in four years: a pandemic, a Parkinson's diagnosis, turning 50. The one thing that remains the same is my love life, which is permanently on hush. What if it stays silent indefinitely? Let's face it: time waits for nobody, which explains my constant fear of being late. I arrive 20 minutes early for dinner reservations, hours before a scheduled flight. I file copy days before a deadline and I once arrived at the dentist a week before my appointment. The irony? Despite my existential anxiety about being left behind, I exhibit a curious nonchalance about big-ticket items like life partners, convinced that what's for me won't pass me by. I'm beginning to think this might be a self-serving bias, a handy cop-out for not putting myself out there. I can't keep waiting for things to be perfect before I make a stab at dating again. Who knows how long that could be? It's far too easy to let life slip away with no one to mark the day. Andy is right. Don't leave it too long.

* * *

Ouch! I jab my finger with a safety pin for the second time this morning. My tremor is quite active and is not helping matters. It must be anticipation nerves. I'm due at Isaac's

Restaurant in two hours for the Parkinson's Fundraising Ladies Lunch and I still need to get to the hairdresser. Hoisting up the waistband of my trousers (which is about two inches too big), I make another stab at securing the excess fabric. *So much for trying these on two weeks ago. How much weight did I lose?* I do a mental risk assessment before making the final call. *What if the safety pin pops open and I stab myself in the waist? Or worse, what if I have to pee? And I always have to pee.* Do I risk self-harm with a wayward clasp, or do I let the trousers hang loose and get my heel caught in the hem when I walk? As I am co-hosting the charity lunch and fashion show, I don't relish falling on my face in front of 150 people, but I don't have the time to change either. Safety pin it is. I put on the matching blazer over my extra small camisole, which is now extra loose. *At least the jacket is oversized* – deliberate or otherwise.

My cab arrives. I shimmy into the back seat, praying the safety pin stays in place, and soon enough we're pulling up in front of what was once a Victorian tobacco factory. Facing the front door of the now fine-dining venue are safety barriers cordoning off MacCurtain Street's never-ending roadworks. Kangos jumping. Concrete breaking. *Clackity! Clackity! Clack!* Why today of all days? Praying the restaurant has some sort of soundproofing, I follow the pedestrian signs onto the footpath and steel myself for a jump scare from the drilling.

Inside, we tick boxes and do double checks before our guests arrive. Soon, the music and the bubbling tempo of chat will sublimate our worries. The soundman hands me a microphone for a *one-two-one-two*. Conscious of my softer register, I lean closer to its steel mesh grille and, unawares, in doing so stand closer to the speaker. As I count, a piercing screech nearly perforates my eardrums and those around me. Great start.

Would-be wardrobe malfunction and potential deafening aside, the afternoon runs smoothly.

In between the fashion show and lunch, I chat to those who took time out of their day to attend. After meeting people at various stages of the disease, it is an apt reminder to avoid overthinking or focusing on things outside of my control. One woman, not much older than me, whose gait instability requires her to use a walking frame, also suffers from decreased speech intelligibility. That means she spends several days a week in speech therapy to make herself understood. How frustrating must that be? Not that she shows it. Sporting a chic blunt bob and silk wrap dress, surrounded by a gaggle of friends, she lives her life without apologies. I think back to the early days of my diagnosis and how I avoided big events, not wanting Parkinson's as a plus one. All of that missing out. Not anymore.

A tap on the microphone and an "excuse me" later, our numbers girl from CUH Charity confirms that we have hit our target of €20,000. The proceeds will go to support the needs of Parkinson's patients at Cork University Hospital's neurology department through CUH Charity. Amazed at people's generosity, I head home with hope in my heart and a sense of achievement. By this time the drills have stopped, of course.

* * *

Ping. That evening, the group chat gets another text from Andy. He's getting a new machine to help him cough, keep his lungs clear and reduce the chance of infection. The MND clinic will provide any support he needs, but the disease is spreading quickly. There are no words. "I'm so sorry," doesn't cut it, especially when someone is barely able to breathe and needs strangers to help them use the toilet. Shamefully, that's all I can muster despite the anger I feel for Andy – angry that he doesn't have the privilege of choice; angry this wretched disease is taking his dignity; angry that soon he won't be able to 'mark the day' as he does every June 7th with dancing, wine and laughter. Mostly, I'm angry with myself for being so insensitive. My friend is dying, yet I make a point of not celebrating my birthday, and *he* sends *me* flowers? Rather than count my blessings, I'm counting wrinkles and regrets.

That Saturday, I'm on the cover of the *Irish Examiner*'s *Weekend* magazine. *What 50 looks like now: Annmarie O'Connor is rewriting the middle-age style rules.* Smiling in jeans and a T-shirt, I look like I don't have a care in the world. And I don't. My medication is finally working. I have my sparkle back. When I do count my blessings, several are missing, but I dare not complain. Good girls don't do that. Instead, I stifle my screams with platitudes and put my pain in a box marked 'later'. Then I tell the universe to go fuck herself.

The following week, an ambulance takes Andy to Our Lady's Hospice in Harold's Cross, his new home.

CHAPTER EIGHT
Side Effects
Here we go again

June 2023

I WAKE UP EVERY morning at 5.30 a.m. This is a recent phenomenon. It used to take a bouncer and an act of God to extract me from the bed, now I don't even need an alarm. Eyes open. Brain active. Feet on the floor. If my calculations are correct, this is largely due to the medication I started four months ago. Why, I don't know. Nor do I understand why, at precisely 9 a.m., I experience 30 minutes of acute anxiety. My heartbeat quickens. I start pacing the floor. The familiar absence makes its presence felt. This is my body preparing me for the surge. Inexplicable sadness and panic take over until I can't catch my breath. I start sobbing, not knowing why but knowing it will pass. And so it goes, every morning. I know the drill by now. Still, it doesn't make it less difficult; having to stay inside my apartment until the turbulence subsides, fearful of having an episode in public.

I make an appointment to speak to the CUH Parkinson's nurse. She is incredibly empathetic. Anxiety is common for people with Parkinson's, especially in the early stages. It's helpful to know that. My upbeat tone suggests this is a minor inconvenience, not a major disruption. I can handle it. But I can't. Why else would I be calling? I know there's no right way of doing Parkinson's, yet my default is always that of an A-student: keen to learn, to please others, to be the best.

We discuss different modalities that might help, like yoga, mindfulness and meditation. Although I have these practices in my toolkit, they are rusty from lack of use. That says it all. Instead, I negotiate adding a few extra hills to my daily walks, which is a manageable ask, especially in Cork. We laugh. Before hanging up, my voice breaks. She notices. I withdraw, feeling embarrassed, playing down my vulnerability. I'm fine. Really. I am. Only I'm not.

Over the next few weeks, my 9 a.m. scaries get scarier. A half hour becomes an hour. Moments of trepidation appear like spectres during the day. I spend a small fortune on CBD gummies, which have no effect. Walking is the one thing that soothes my mood, so I increase my daily target from 10,000 to 15,000 steps. Some days, I do more. I still feel anxious, but in lieu of waiting for it to pass, I walk around the apartment while watching mindless reality TV on my phone. Pacing up and down the hallway is weirdly calming yet requires a degree of conscious awareness so as not to walk into a wall or clip a door frame, which I am apt to do. Plus, the regular dose of celebrity schadenfreude is a tonic of the 'could be worse' variety.

Committing to a regular exercise routine helps take my mind off my mind. Soon, I find myself applying this self-same consistency to my diet, treating my body like a proverbial temple rather than a garden shed: homemade soups, healthy salads, lean protein, lots of water, no alcohol, no sweet food apart from the occasional treat. I'm especially particular about food timings and doing what I can to ensure optimal medication absorption. My A-student is calling the shots. She's a hard worker, but, my God, she's also hard work.

* * *

Julie and I are meeting for coffee at the shopping centre. It's a gem of a day: 24 degrees Celsius and sunny with a warm breeze, not a cloud in the sky. I'm wearing jeans and a Merino wool sweater. In Ireland, this is considered treason. It's like flipping the bird to Mother Nature. Usually, she throws everything at us: sheet rain, sideways wind, mutant hailstones. Our bar is so low when it comes to decent weather that we sea swim in winter for fun. I'm cold though and a bit tired, so jeans and a sweater it is.

Julie is waiting for me at the café when I arrive, all smiles and hellos, the usual. Except it's not. Julie's face is etched with worry. Something is up.

We order two Americanos. I don't have cake.

I tell her about my recent visit to Andy in hospice. It's all I can think about. "Two weeks of respite," he said and then he can go home, but even that looks uncertain. "He was barely able to speak to me, Jules."

"I can't begin to imagine how hard that must be for you, seeing him like that and not being able to do anything to help him. I'm so sorry."

Julie's "sorry" feels like an emotional support blanket. I wrap each syllable around my heart. I know what's coming.

"Annie, you've lost weight again." I nod in agreement. "Your legs – they look so tiny."

My relationship with food is a touchy subject. Julie remembers. "It's not like college," I reassure her, explaining that although my appetite is increasing, so has my daily exercise to help mitigate symptoms like anxiety.

"Promise me you'll look after yourself." And I do promise. Not wanting to spoil our chat, I ask her how she's settling into the new house.

"The place needs a lot of work," she admits. "I feel like I have things under control, except for the blasted Wi-Fi, which I need to sort out now before my children go mad."

After Julie leaves, I head to Dunnes Stores to buy a bathroom scales. I don't typically engage with numbers. It's not healthy for me. Having always been a UK size 12, I have an idea of my weight, but after seeing Julie's look of concern, I need proof.

Later on, I'm standing in my underwear, wondering if this is a good idea. If I step on the scales, I'll know like I know. *You're a 50-year-old woman,* I remind myself. And so, I step up. The LCD reads 136 pounds. I'm in shock. I step off the glass surface and try again. One hundred and thirty-six pounds. I grab my phone and ask Google: *Are digital scales more accurate than manual ones?* They are, but that's not the point. Julie is right. I have lost a lot of weight, but a part of me wonders if a small part of me wants this.

* * *

I doze off at my desk, head lolling, arms flopping like a limp marionette. I'm not out for long, just until my neck smarts from the dead weight.

Thirty minutes later, it happens again.

That evening, I'm doing some research for a creative pitch. I make a pot of coffee, sit in my hard-backed chair and conk out for an hour.

Excessive daytime sleepiness (EDS) is a side effect of the dopaminergic medications used to treat Parkinson's, which I take several times a day. That makes falling prey to an impromptu snooze highly likely. Dopamine also regulates saliva production, so, to make things interesting, there's drool. No warning. No "here it comes!" Nothing an intravenous coffee drip or open window in winter can ever fix. What's more, these moments invariably happen when I'm comfortably seated before my laptop, the fan humming its ASMR lullaby.

As a result, I'm not getting much done. Instead, I am surrounded by ideas in their infancy, semi-started projects and half-filled carts waiting in virtual checkouts. It's concerning. When I'm not asleep on the job, I'm prone to flash naps: eyes wide open, no facial expression, no words – just a five-second 404 error. Patricia, who's visiting me in Cork this week with my niece, is the only person who seems to spot and stop these episodes.

"You're doing it again."

No response.

Patricia leans across the table and clicks her fingers. "Ams, snap out of it."

I emerge from the glitch in the matrix, semi-startled. We chuckle as I shake my head in mild embarrassment. "Sorry, Trish!"

"I was mid-story about Rosie when I noticed you weren't with us."

"At least I didn't fall asleep on you," I admit. "That's my new schtick. It's probably the meds, but I made an appointment with my GP next week for routine blood work. With the weight loss and the tiredness, I want to put my mind at rest. Plus, the constant overthinking is taking its toll."

"Good. I'm glad you're on top of it. I told you ages ago that you were getting too thin." Patricia is a pioneer of firsts:

the first to notice, to say something, to do something about the something that was said that she noticed ages before anyone else thought to say something. I could never accuse her of apathy. Not ever.

As with Julie, I tell her it's a combination of things, but mainly a side effect of the medication. Before I can continue, her early-warning radar detects something. "When did you get the scales in the bathroom?" Her casual tone is disarming.

"A few days ago. I met Julie for coffee in the village. She was worried about how thin I've got, so I bought one to find out what I weigh." I pause. "It's not deliberate. Not this time."

The past fills the space between us.

"I'm 136 pounds, Trish."

Not one to tarry, Patricia presents an interim solution. "When you see your GP next week, ask if she can put you on a nutritional supplement like Complan. Nursing homes often use it for people who lose their appetites." I tell her I will, but that small part of me wants no part of it. I don't tell her that. Instead, I change the subject to plans for this evening: dinner reservations in the village at 8 p.m.

"The water is hot for showers," I say with camp counsellor enthusiasm, setting the tone for the rest of the evening and I excuse myself to get changed. Forty minutes later, I'm still not ready. I look at the pile of discarded clothes on my bed. *There has to be something that looks half-decent.* Dressing a body that once felt like home can be an isolating experience. I am a squatter with no rights to this partial land: void contours and absent curves, strong headlands of muscle now barren. Nothing is familiar.

I make a snap decision and go for my black knit midi dress, which covers the saggy skin on my knees and thighs. Unconvinced, I slip on a pair of ballet flats and do one last outfit check before joining the others on the balcony. *I'm pretty sure this is as good as it gets,* I guess.

We take a group selfie before mercifully walking downhill on what happens to be the longest day of the year. As we're about to leave, I ask Patricia to take a quick picture of me for my Instagram Stories. "Gotta feed the algorithm before we get fed!"

"Well, in that case, say 'chicken burger'," she exclaims, knowing I've already stalked the menu. Handing me back the phone, I scroll through the shots as she grabs my house keys. "Don't forget these," she reminds me with a knowing look. Not that I'm paying attention. I fixate on my bony arms, gaunt face and protruding veins. *Is this how others see me? Maybe it's a bad camera angle.* I debate whether to post the photo online. *Don't overthink it. It's just Instagram.* My thumb hovers over the 'Your Story' button. I press. I post. I delete it later that evening, changing the narrative.

* * *

Stick or twist? Right now, there are two piles of clothes on my bed: what fits and what doesn't. I make a third, otherwise I'll be very cold and possibly incarcerated for indecent exposure. It is a 'let's see' pile: my sartorial escrow for a time in the future yet undetermined. When decluttering wardrobes, I usually only recommend the third pile if a client is experiencing significant ongoing change – a bit like me. Waiting for the dust to settle and getting things back on track seems contradictory, but so is life: moving into a house when the paint is barely dry, going back to work after burying a family member, or dating while navigating a messy divorce.

The binary 'keep or let go' philosophy of traditional wardrobe clearouts greatly benefits from a third pile: the opportunity to reflect before making any big decisions while still dressing the person you are today. At the heart of my current 'closet full of clothes and nothing to wear' conundrum is change. No one is immune. We often undergo the same challenges at different junctures in our lives until we learn the lesson. Trust me, this is not my first rodeo.

I try on a few of my vintage dresses for size. Most of them are from my favourite era, the 1970s, and they include an Adele Simpson floral maxi dress and a similar anonymous beauty I imagine once belonged to a South Beach socialite. All that's missing is a Martini – three olives, dirty, no twist.

Sadly, my body has lost its hanger appeal. When Patricia and I go to Inishbofin next month, I'll ask Mom about altering them. Maybe she can take in a few of them for me when she comes to visit next. Back to my predicament. What the hell do I wear *now*? The fact is, a shopping trip is in order before I make any culls. All I need are a few stopgap staples that fit whether I gain or lose more weight: a drawstring waist here and a bit of stretch there. For the time being, I'm sticking with online shopping. Inconvenient as it might be, I don't fancy someone knocking on my dressing room door asking if everything is OK when I am forced to take an honest look in the mirror.

July 2023

A few weeks later, Patricia is driving us to Cleggan to take the Inishbofin ferry. The weather is unruly as usual: spitting rain and wind chill that leaves bite marks. Poor Mom – anytime we visit, she might as well put the barbecue in the shed. We need our auras cleansed or, at the very least, a few Child of Prague statues in the boot of the car.

"It feels good knowing what's ahead," I muse, watching the Twelve Bens grow in the distance. "By the way, I got my results—"

"Did you remember to buy those acupressure bands?"

"Yes, but can I finish what I was saying?"

"Sorry, just while I thought of it."

She shoots me an apologetic smile. "Menopause brain."

"So, yeah. I got my results from my—"

"I just had a vision of having to carry your limp body onto the pier. I already threw my back out cleaning the shower this week."

To be fair, these panic-filled interruptions are not for nothing. I once got motion sick in Patricia's new car. Correction: I once got motion-sick *all over* Patricia's new car. After a few too many bumps down country roads, I vomited ad nauseum into a plastic bag I found in the glove compartment. Before she had time to pull over so I could bin the offending item, the anti-suffocation hole split and the bag burst open onto my trousers. So, that happened. Now that I can't take motion sickness tablets, there are two of us who are a bit twitchy.

She apologises. "Go on, you were saying . . ."

I tidy up my interrupted thoughts and continue, "So, I got my results from my GP. I have low ferritin and low B12, which also explains my sleepiness. I requested an iron infusion on account of my slow gut, and I've already started my course of B12 shots. She's also organising a gastroscopy and colonoscopy to be on the safe side. There might be an absorption issue I'm not aware of. On that note, I've arranged to see a Parkinson's dietitian, too."

"Good on you, missus. I'm delighted. You won't know yourself in a month or so. Have you spoken to the physio yet about your shoulder?"

After 15 years of schlepping garment bags, cases and industrial-sized steamers up elevators, down steps, on trains, through traffic, across the country and back again, my right shoulder is giving me grief. Years of neglect coupled with Parkinson's have resulted in osteoarthritis and a bang of tendonitis. Having lost weight, the lack of cushioning and depleted muscle mass around my clavicle, AC joint and forearm now makes anything load bearing an act of self-harm. In fact, my shoulder and I are not on speaking terms unless you count expletives when applying Deep Heat.

"I'm heading to CUH before the bank holiday. In the meantime, I'm using a backpack to ease the pressure." I can tell Patricia is amused. Backpacks are not my preferred aesthetic, but neither is crippling pain. "You should try one of those mobility trollies."

I recoil in horror at the very suggestion. "I think you're making a mountain out of a molehill."

"I think you're wrong. Most people need a nebuliser getting up that incline from the bus stop to your apartment."

My ego has a meltdown while Patricia sells me the features and benefits of wheeled carryalls. "There are lovely leopard print ones on DoneDeal – waterproof too."

"I'm sure there are, but I'd sooner consent to having my colonoscopy administered by a hot doctor before using one of those, lovely leopard print or otherwise."

The following week, my physio proffers similar advice: no totes, no oversized shoppers, no gargantuan suitcases. Thankfully, she does not include emotional baggage, which would require a light cargo plane. But I digress.

With my AC now RIP, I have two options: a light crossbody or a wheelable shopping trolley, favoured by savvy seniors and, of course, my sister Patricia.

Small is not my strong suit. As a stylist, my bag requirements hinge on the premise "If it can't fit a bottle of wine, some boob tape, a ring light and a portable wind machine, why have one?" Don't get me wrong, I like the ease and lack of schedule that something petite implies, but I have a tough enough time filling an airport security Ziploc without breaking out in a sweat. As for the trolley? I need time to consider my options – about another 20 years or so.

August 2023

Ping.

"God only knows what they could find up there . . . a Chanel clutch bag, one of your crystals, a bottle of Prosecco . . ."

"That doesn't sound so bad, to be honest!"

I'm in the waiting room, texting Neil before my endoscopy. For clarification, it involves a tube with a camera being inserted in your throat and again in your back passage, usually when unexplained weight loss or digestive symptoms present. Plus, you get to watch the drama unfold as it happens on a widescreen TV. Good times. I suspect the lack of dopamine in my brain is starting to rewire my definition of entertainment.

I'm choosing conscious sedation for today's proceedings, which comes with a few caveats. Forbidden for the next 24 hours are things like taking a taxi, working out, cooking, drinking alcohol, operating heavy machinery – and being alone without a responsible adult. No chaperone. No discharge. No dice.

Filling out the admission form, I tell a half lie by saying that I will be signed out by a responsible adult with whom I will stay for 24 hours. It's a flawed premise. How can you assess the degree to which someone is responsible? By taking my word for it after conscious sedation? That's not wise.

Back in 2015, I thought I spotted Joe Dolan at Dublin Pride. Neil and Andy kindly informed me that although our national treasure lives in our hearts, he is indeed dead and has been for several years. Ditto for Mick Lally. It just so happens that Julie is a paragon of responsibility. Of course, if anyone asks, I'm spending the night at her house.

Once the receptionist calls my name, I am prepped and ready for theatre in minutes. There's a sense of mild urgency in the air, as if the doctor has to pick up the kids from GAA practice and wants to avoid the work traffic. Two nurses escort me across the hall to the theatre as I wrestle with the open-back paper gown. *Not exactly Met Gala material but neither is today's agenda.*

I prop myself onto the cold metal table, a request made by a tall voice in blue scrubs. The voice turns around. *Are you kidding me? Wait until Patricia finds out.* It's my hot doctor (marital status pending), also known as Dr Smith. While briefing me on the first procedure, he sprays the back of my throat with a numbing solution and administers the conscious sedation. The next ten minutes are a fever dream of sorts: coughing, spluttering, convinced of my untimely death. Four years of regular yoga practice and breathing exercises do not prepare a gag reflex for that ordeal. Then the good stuff kicks in – pure liquid confidence.

For the second procedure, I lean on my side with my head in my hand, watching my colon in all its HD glory. "So, doctor, what are we looking at here?" I am blatantly flirting with a highly qualified stranger who is currently inserting a tube up my bottom. A first, I'll admit. Graciously, he talks me through my intestinal tract while I tell him about my Parkinson's and how today nearly didn't happen.

"That liquid laxative didn't work until I took the second dose. I set up vigil in my bathroom with *Below Deck* on my laptop. Four episodes of season seven later and there was still no motion in the ocean. It's crazy what low dopamine can do." Once the endoscopy is over, he reassures me there is nothing sinister going on and gives me the all clear. An hour in the recovery ward and I am free to go.

"With my responsible adult," I chime in. "Her name is Julie. She's my best friend." You see? Always the A-student, even when under the influence. "Thanks a million, doctor." I wave, still talking, as my gurney retreats into the hallway. I briefly chat to the orderly who brings me tea and toast, but apart from that, I'm on my tod and feeling remarkably social. *God, I'm dying for a chat.* One of the cleaners pops in to wipe down the empty beds beside me.

"Where are you from?" I ask. "Do you like your job? Things must have been tough during COVID."

Words, words, words. All the words. Here they are. All at once. All for you. More words.

Julie arrives in time to save the man, who looks immeasurably relieved.

I gather my things, still talking: "So, yeah. That's why I changed my health insurance," while she signs the release form for the nurse on duty. Guiding me by my elbow, Julie co-pilots me out of the ward and, like an award-winning actor, I thank everyone on the way out. Everyone.

"How did you get on?" she asks as we make our way to the car park.

"Oh, I've got the all clear. More importantly, the doctor was *so* hot but *so* married. I managed to crane my head and spot his ring before we got ... familiar, shall we say. Whatever sedative he gave me, I feel like it's Friday night and we're back living in London," I reminisce. "It's that lovely getting-ready feeling: a combination of expectation and promise. The world was our oyster. I miss that." My feet begin to feel heavy as the effects of Friday night wear off.

Julie pats my hand. "You'll sleep tonight, Annie."

"Eight hours of unconscious sedation with any luck."

"Now, *that* sounds like a great night."

* * *

Dr Sweeney is leaving. I just found out, and I'm gutted. He reassures me that my new consultant is top-notch. When I meet her, I understand why. I'm in great hands, but the handover makes me realise how much trust you can place in one person. It really is a leap of faith, especially weighing up the immediacy of medication and its possible side effects while getting your head and heart around operations like deep brain stimulation or needing a carer down the line. Although quality of life is quantifiable in medical terms, our lived experience is mutable and often at odds with the blind spot of expectation. It's common to think that taking three tablets a day will help manage Parkinson's symptoms. It's also common to get despondent when they don't. Neither is wrong, so long as we learn to recalibrate any existing assumptions in line with what we now know. That's growth. Mindset shifts are not easy, that I know. Why else would we be creatures of habit? Having someone who understands these constant moving parts – both physical and psychological – is a gift. Here's to you, Dr Sweeney. You'll be missed.

* * *

I'm starting my five-day food diary for the Parkinson's dietitian. One more box to tick and that's me done for the summer. Honestly, I'm wrecked. Between GP visits and hospital, physio and outpatient appointments, I am using all my free time to catch up on work. As a result, my meticulously lined bullet journal, designated for tracking my steps, medication and symptoms, remains conspicuously empty. Replacing its contents are voice-to-text notes on my phone and codified shorthand that even I can't understand. Sometimes life gets in the way, but I must remember it's my life and it's all I've got. So, I best treat it accordingly.

The purpose of this diary is to determine if certain foods trigger my symptoms or whether it's the timing of my medication relative to my meals and snacks. To that end, I must record everything, from the amount I eat, sleep and exercise to my hydration and perceived stress levels. Usually, I am quite disciplined in planning and cooking my meals, but last week's endoscopy put the kibosh on that with its preparation involving a three-day, low-residue diet featuring nothing but beige food: white toast, mashed potato, cottage cheese, Rice Krispies and everyone's favourite, water biscuits. It's like the bland apocalypse. You'll die of boredom before the zombies ever get to you. Note to self: I should remember to organise my Tesco delivery *before* claiming I eat well and recording evidence to the contrary.

Part of me wants to delay the exercise until my shelves are stocked with fresh fruit, vegetables and lean meats. It feels like I'm agreeing to take a test for which I haven't studied. Still, in the interest of transparency, I'll fully commit to the exercise. It will be helpful to understand what I'm lacking energy-wise and to gain some feedback on my overall health. Plus, I could also use advice on timing food and medication, which can be challenging. In other words, I cheat if I get too hungry. Not often, though. Otherwise, I feel like I'm cheating myself. That's my A-student again, calling the shots.

* * *

My kitchen table is special. When friends and family visit, I dress it with woven placemats, hammered gold flatware and hand-painted cloth napkins rolled in jute holders. If the occasion calls for it, I'll elevate stemmed glasses on marble coasters and illuminate a floral centrepiece with tea lights. For me, setting the table is more than a decorative act, it signifies the importance of spending time together: a shared experience through food.

I adhere to this practice even when I eat alone, holding space for a proper meal at least once a day. When I lose respect for the ritual, I lose respect for myself. I am no longer accountable for the health of my body.

My A-student starts policing what I eat, allowing me half of something and throwing out the rest. Never satisfied, I hover at the fridge, taking small mouthfuls of this and that. *Cop on. Be more disciplined*, she says. Caught between the polarities of too much and not enough, she enforces self-appointed rules at will: no eating between meals, before medication doses or after certain hours. It gets tiring. That's when I set the table less. There comes a point where I don't even bother. The table is bare.

Not anymore. Today, the table is set. Julie is coming round for afternoon tea after she feeds the kids which is, by the sound of the front doorbell, sooner than expected.

I hear speech- and drama-trained pronunciation from the hallway. "It's only me. Downstairs was unlocked."

"That's what the last cult recruiter said. Now, please leave before I call the police."

I open the door, still buckled from my not-so-funny joke. Julie, meanwhile, spots the tablescaping, completely missing her hug and "hello, darling" cue.

"Annie, you outdid yourself. It's Martha Stewart level, and what's this?" she exclaims, pointing to a three-tier confectionary stand.

"Oh, that's made from Mom and Dad's wedding dinnerware. Rather than it be given to one of us, Margaret had a little something made for all of us."

The tower of crustless sandwiches and mini scones begins to wobble. So does my heart, which is currently in my mouth.

"I went a little over the top," I admit, removing a few unsteady goodies. "With the kids back in school this week, I thought it would be a nice treat to mark the end of the summer."

Happy to play host, I pour tea and portion out ramekins of clotted cream and jam to the light riffs of soft jazz. I have something else to share. Something important, but it can wait. Rather than drop a home truth on her plate the moment she sits down, I allow Julie to lead the conversation, feeding her question after question.

"That's enough about me," she insists as if she's been overserved. "So, tell me, how are you doing?" She leans on her clasped hands, eager to hear my news. I offer an unconvincing "grand" before delivering a report on my rather prosaic food diary for the Parkinson's dietitian.

"The results show that I am not meeting my energy requirements. In addition to the significant lack of calories, my diet is low on healthy fats, carbohydrates, B vitamins, iron, iodine, selenium and zinc, which might be playing into my anxiety."

"I'm so embarrassed," I confess. "The word 'malnutrition' was used. I've been deluding myself that I eat well, not realising I am part of the problem."

"By 'well' do you mean 'disciplined'?" Julie asks. I nod.

"And the problem being . . .?"

"It's quite common for people with Parkinson's to lose weight when trying to manage medications and food timings."

Julie knows this isn't the actual reason. She waits for me to catch up.

"It started after the injection trial in January. When that treatment didn't work, I leaned into diet and exercise to maintain some control over my Parkinson's symptoms. A month and a half later, the patch completely transformed my world for the better, short of the initial appetite loss. Somewhere along the way, though, the lines got blurred. I got thinner, but I was also starting to feel better. Maybe I conflated the two, but I liked how I felt until it began to feel way too familiar – like it did in college."

Julie remembers.

"I don't want to go back there. It was hard enough recognising I had a problem." My lip starts to quiver. "I remember sitting alone and crying at the kitchen table in our college flat, making myself eat, knowing I had to. Because I never sought treatment, I had no idea how to navigate that point in my life. To this day, I find it difficult to say I had an eating disorder. I don't feel I own it."

"And yet here you are, getting ahead of it. I'm so proud of you."

"It's just very triggering to be experiencing something again that I thought was over." Julie looks at the untouched scone on my plate.

"It's never really over, though, is it, Annie? Things get better, but sometimes the past comes back to be healed."

"Come to think of it, Mercury is in Retrograde now in the sign of Virgo. It's all about inward reflection, self-analysis and addressing old wounds so that we meet our full potential."

"I always thought you hated Mercury Retrograde." Julie knows I'm an astrology apologist.

"Oh, I don't love it, that's for sure. Communication is challenging. Things can feel like they're going backwards but not without reason, especially if you take the time to reflect, revisit or redo things. I've come so far. I don't want to go backwards, Jules."

"You're not," she smiles, grabbing my hand. "You just took a detour."

"And to think, I'm always the one to harp on about no right way of doing Parkinson's, which is just as well given the balls I've made of it."

I laugh at myself while wiping away a tear.

"Life is messy, Annie."

"It is," I reply, casting a glance over the chinoiserie plates and matching teacups. There's a crack in one of them.

"Jules . . . I'm afraid of how I'll feel when I start gaining weight again. I never did close that chapter from college."

"Maybe now's the time."

CHAPTER NINE
Full Circle
Lessons learned

September 2023

LIFE'S UNCONVENTIONAL MOMENTS ARE often more entertaining than the highlights on which we fixate. This occurs to me as I write another post for my new Substack blog: *Wanted: A Responsible Adult*. Its titular inspiration stems from the shenanigans surrounding my recent endoscopy and, by extension, the absurd minutiae of my world. I use it to keep my creative writing fresh and to document these seemingly inconsequential happenings. Now I'm eating my words. Open in a separate laptop window is an email from the editor of *Irish Tatler* inviting me to an event I'll never forget. It goes something like this:

> I'm sending you a quick note as we've just finished judging the Women of the Year 2023 Awards. You have been shortlisted for the Catalyst category, which recognises women affecting social change in Irish society. Would you be free on 11th November to attend the event in The Shelbourne? It's a spangly affair but it's also about celebrating amazing

women doing brilliant things, which you are! Love it if you could be there. An official invitation is on its way.

This is big. So big that I let out an exclamatory squeal. Curious to discover more about the event, I look back at previous winners online across categories that include media, STEM, music and public life and I feel humbled, if not sceptical. Are they sure I'm on the shortlist? Maybe it's an admin error? Or I'm just overthinking my way out of a lovely moment. I reply to the editor with effusive thanks, ensuring her I will be there. She tells me I can bring a plus one, so I immediately text Neil and ask him to be my date. It's time that I celebrate myself or, as Andy says, to 'mark the day'. This is not a mistake. This is happening. I couldn't be happier.

* * *

"Bring those dresses to me, dear, along with your mending kit. I'll have that sorted in no time." Mom is visiting me in Cork and offering to alter my special vintage pieces. Her dressmaking ability, even without a sewing machine, is bang-on accurate.

As a kid, I remember her sitting at the kitchen table with a pin cushion around her wrist and a stitch pick in her hand. "That woman paid good money for this skirt," she'd gripe, explaining the importance of a decent seam allowance. Then there was Nana, who'd side-eye a stranger's jumper in the name of quality control, "No double-blind stitches on that hem," she'd say out of earshot, shaking her head with mild contempt. "That's a sin, you know."

"Ams!" I hear Mom calling me.

"Dear, this is as far as I can alter it without compromising the shape of the dress." She holds up a 1970s jacquard knit gown with fluted sleeves – one of my favourites. "I can take it home and recut it for you based on your measurements, but you've gone down about two sizes already."

"No worries. I'll try it on and we can decide then," I say, my arms wrapped around my fleece robe as I try to keep warm.

"Dear, you're freezing," she says, bunching the dress's fabric like an accordion so that I can slip it on over my head. That's Mom-code for "something is wrong".

Worried she'll spot my protruding ribs, I offer to step into it instead and, doing so, deflect from a potentially awkward moment.

The fabric dangles from my frame. I don't consult the mirror.

"I tell you what," Mom suggests with gusto. "How about I take them home with me. This way I can work on them at my machine and send them back to you by registered post."

"It's OK, Mom. I like a looser fit, anyway. Besides, I'll be thankful for the extra room when I gain back a bit of weight."

The look on Mom's face says she wish she could do more. Mine too.

"Honestly, don't worry. I just thought it would be handy not to have to buy something new."

"What about the Women of the Year Awards?"

"Not a problem. I'm going to visit Andy in Dublin next week. I'll have that sorted in no time."

October 2023

I am in Dublin for a press event – my first in a long time – and to see Andy. "You're lucky," Neil tells me over the phone. "He's enforcing a visitor embargo now. Each time he uses the breathing support tube to help him speak, it sets him back a few paces the following day. His energy levels just aren't up to it." We plan to meet at the hospice later that afternoon as Neil has a work call. That gives Andy and me time to catch up. I arrive around 3.30 p.m., bag in hand containing aromatherapy room spray and tubs of mini bites from M&S. He is in his wheelchair, which is kitted out with a hands-free eye gaze control screen. I'm so happy to see him and, all things being equal, he's looking well.

"Hey, handsome!" I smile and kiss him on the cheek before I unbag his treats on the adjacent table. He gestures for me to pass him the breathing apparatus on the bedside locker.

"Jesus, Andy, this thing looks like a vape," I remark. He puts it between his hands, inhales deeply and begins to hold court, just like that day on the Eames chair.

"You've lost weight."

"Well, don't waste time. Get to the point," I joke.

He takes another hit.

"You're not eating."

"I am."

And another.

"Not enough."

And again.

It worries me that Andy is using his valuable breath to tell me off. A hit from the breathing support tube usually lasts him a few sentences, not just a few words.

"You're right. I am a bit thin," I admit, preferring to concede defeat so as not to wear him out.

A knock on the door interrupts my interrogation as a nurse drops off a plate of lasagne and chips on her rounds.

"Hungry?"

Andy nods.

"You must be starving because you never let me feed you," I wink, lifting the dome-shaped cover with a mischievous shake.

"If you do wind up with half the dinner down your chin, please accept my apologies in advance." Chatting about pure nonsense while expertly keeping equal parts of pasta, veg and mince on each forkful, I surpass my expectations and Andy's – much to his relief, I'm sure. I even go so far as to feed him one of the chocolate millionaires to finish the meal, which he tries and dismisses. The mini flapjacks are the star buy, both of us agree. Taking a seat on the bed opposite his chair, we return to our usual programming. This time he notices how well my medication is working and asks me about the upcoming Women of the Year Awards. When Neil arrives, the energy shifts and a healthy dose of banter ensues. It's like old times – the same but different.

Before we know it, it's time to leave. "We'd better get going if you want to make that 6 p.m. train," Neil advises. "I've got to head back to work for a bit. Traffic is brutal." We say our goodbyes to Andy, warm ones filled with laughter, and as per Neil's prediction, wind up in gridlock for an hour. I miss my train by five minutes, only to discover the second one is late due to a bridge strike in Portlaoise. I spend the next two hours in Heuston station fending off entitled pigeons and listening to Tannoy updates beginning with "We are sorry to announce . . ." By the time I get home, it's 11 p.m. I feel shattered but satisfied. There is a sense of completion about the day that I can't describe: the three of us hanging out together and putting the world to rights – the usual.

Neil calls me the following evening to check in and to apologise on Andy's behalf.

"The first words out of his mouth when I went to see him today were, 'I think I offended Ams.' He basically ratted on himself."

"Oh!" I start to giggle, recalling Andy's hatred of censorship.

"Before you went to see him on Thursday, I specifically said, 'Ams has lost a lot of weight. She's very sensitive right now. Please don't mention it.'"

"It's fine," I reassure him. "I know he meant well, judging by the strength he needed just to get the words out."

Andy, as we know, is not one for verbiage. In a world filled with blatherskites and confidence men, his blunt delivery is like rubbing alcohol on an open wound: it stings in the moment, but it does the job. I need it to sting occasionally.

"He told me the same thing in April," I note, "only this time, he got straight to the point. It felt like he had things he needed to say. I'm not offended.

"Look," I continue, "while we're on the subject of food, I was asked by *Irish Tatler* if you had any dietary requirements. I said no but I was tempted to declare, 'Your best Champagne, garçon!' If you've become a low-salt, demi-gluten, flexitarian forager since we last spoke, let me know, and they'll put it on your preference sheet."

"Ams, you know I only eat food the same colour as my aura that day," Neil insists. "I also intermittently fast according to the times of the tide. Otherwise, all good."

* * *

It's Saturday. Mom calls me in the morning, after her first cup of coffee and before she changes out of her pyjamas.

"Dear, it's only Mom. I hope I'm not disturbing you."

"Not at all," I say clicking-to-cart. "I'm just shopping for shoes to pair with my dress for the Women of the Year Awards."

"You got the dress? Wow! That was fast."

"I picked it up yesterday from Miss Daisy Blue. It's vintage Oscar de la Renta – a light green metallic brocade with gold piping. The owner kindly let me borrow it along with a 1950s hard-case metallic clutch."

"Make sure you send a photo when you have a moment. I'm dying to see it."

"I'll try it on so you get a better idea. Mom, it fits like a glove, but you know me, I'm sitting here wondering what the catch is. It all feels too easy. For example, I found a pair of UK size nine shoes just now after ten minutes of noodling on the internet. When does that ever happen? Usually, I'm searching high and low, buzzing around, trying to find something for my big feet. *Then* I wind up trading off on what I want to get what I need."

"Dear, you always did worry too much, even as a child. You've got to learn to let things come to you and, when they do, not to question them."

"I think I have blue-arsed fly syndrome."

Mom chortles on the other end. "You always did have a way with words. Speaking of which, have you prepared your speech?"

"What speech?"

"For your award."

"Oh, Mom. I've only been shortlisted."

"Still and all, you should have a few words ready, just in case. Here you are worried about what to wear," she chides. "When you win, you know who to thank."

I laugh. "You have infinite faith in me."

"That I do. You're my daughter first and foremost, and let's not forget the good you've done with the hand you've been dealt. You've given people a voice."

"Thanks, Mom."

"I couldn't be prouder. Now, dear, I better get body and soul together before I turn to seed. *Oof!* Good Lord, when did standing up turn into such an ordeal? Once I get the kinks out, I'm grand, but that requires some finessing at my age. I can't complain though. It's simply gorgeous outside."

"I take it you have plans for the garden."

"Oh, I do, indeed, at least until it gets dark. Now, I best get this show on the road. Bye, dear." Mom's garden is her happy place. Should you be unable to find her, always check the potting shed.

November 11, 2023

"I'm so sorry." The cab driver apologises for the second time. "It's usually not this busy on a weekend. I don't know what the problem is." He rubs his bald spot as if it were a Magic 8 Ball. I tell him I'm in no rush and not to worry. He rubs it again, looking for a different answer. Today's traffic jams, reveals a radio report, are due to a death on the M50: someone took their life on an overlooking bridge. I feel winded. *There's no rush*, I think to myself. *Just relax.*

The journey takes an hour longer than usual, yet we arrive in plenty of time. The driver removes my bags from the boot, still apologising and still stroking his head. "This usually doesn't happen," he reminds me.

Margaret is travelling for work and will be home later this evening, so I use the spare key to let myself in and get situated. I unzip the garment bag, allowing my dress to exhale as I lay out a few more bits and bobs: gold kitten-heel shoes, my dad's Claddagh ring and a pair of antique clip-on earrings from a friend in New York. My hair is already coiffed into a sixties-style ponytail, so there isn't much else to do except get my makeup done. There's enough time to make tea and eat the veggie wrap in my bag. There's enough time to relax. There's no rush. I think of the chat with Mom the other day. It can be this easy . . . if I let it.

Downstairs in the kitchen, I fill up the kettle, find a drawer filled with plates and placemats, and set the table for one. It's quiet, bar the water beginning to boil, so I take the next few minutes to give myself a well-needed morale boost.

Tonight is a night of celebration. Savour it. Don't waste time micromanaging a moment that is already perfect. Let go. Not too much, though. You might have to go on stage. So, easy on the cocktails. What I'm trying to say is life is short. Enjoy yourself. Enjoy this time with Neil. Enjoy marking the day. Most of all, wake up tomorrow morning with stories to tell, not regrets.

Ping. Neil texts me to see if I'm in Dublin yet and to confirm our plan for the evening. I ask him if he can swing by Margaret's place first to help me with my zip and to take a look at the back of my hair.

For a house with so many mirrors, none are full-length, I note, rather mystified. Plus, I wouldn't mind doing a quick run-through of a small speech I prepared. Then we can grab a glass of fizz in the Horseshoe Bar before the event.

Neil gets stuck in unusual traffic, most likely from the fatal incident that afternoon. *There is no rush,* I text him. *We have plenty of time.*

Soon, a bell rings, followed by a knock. I open the door to six-foot-three-inches of handsome standing in a black tux.

"You stone-cold fox. Why are you gay?"

He grabs my hands and gives me a twirl. "Speechless!"

While the mutual admiration society is in session, Neil finishes zipping my dress, gives my ponytail a final check and asks if I have everything I need. Then it hits me.

"Speech! Quick, before we go," I scurry into the living room for an understudy trophy and grab one of the decorative church candles that Mags has on display beside the hearth.

Facing Neil and the invisible crowd, I start by thanking *Irish Tatler*. Then, without warning, my tremor throws a diva strop and decides it's her night. Things get a bit wobbly.

Neil laughs out of pure nerves. "Jesus, girl. Whatever you do, don't drop it."

"Come to think of it, I did see a magpie this morning and never waved." Superstitions never fail to get the better of me.

"Oh, that would be it for sure," he jibes. "Nothing to do with your L-dopa wearing off or the fact that you can't walk two feet in Dublin without seeing one of those winged scavengers."

I somehow manage to remember my speech between Neil's friendly fire and my unintentional body movements. We take a few standard-issue selfies for posterity before calling a cab. I grab my coat and bag from upstairs, turn off the landing light and set the house alarm. Fifteen seconds of beeping counts us down.

"OK, mister. Are you ready to have the night of your life?"

"Only if you are."

* * *

Seated under the domed ceilings of the grand ballroom at the Shelbourne Hotel, the event begins with the first of 18 categories: STEM. The editor of *Irish Tatler* shares a short personal biography of the first nominee before inviting her on stage to accept the award. I wonder why the other nominees have not been announced, until the next category follows suit. Neil and I look at each other. "It's either a *very* short shortlist, or you're the Catalyst winner," he whispers. I scan the running order to discover my category is 17th – the penultimate award before the overall winner is announced. "Well, no wine for me, so."

I try to stay in the moment and absorb these incredible stories of the trailblazing women impacting Irish society. *What ifs* interrupt the flow of the evening, from forgetting my speech to falling out of my tad-too-big shoes.

The *what-ifs* win. *Jesus, I'm nervous.* Neil spots it.

"Relax, Ams. People will start asking you to blink twice if you need help. Remember: this is your night." He smiles, and I blink twice for funsies.

"I'm sure you know this, but it was this day last year when you spoke to Tommy Tiernan about a very uncertain future. And yet, despite that, you carried yourself with gumption and positivity. Your story is your superpower. It gives others the licence to tell theirs. Those aren't my words. They're yours. Check your speech."

He points to my phone on the white tablecloth.

"You've come so far since then. Think of it as a full-circle moment." I start to unclench and take a sip of water.

"Promise me a glass of rosé later?"

"Consider it done."

Time flies despite there being no rush. Before long, the editor announces the Catalyst category. "New-York-born, Cork-based Annmarie O'Connor has had much success in her life as an author, editor and stylist . . ."

This is it. Let the good things come to you.

"In August 2022, O'Connor wrote a column with a very different subject matter at its heart. She penned, for the first time, about her experience of being diagnosed with early-onset Parkinson's disease in her forties. This was followed by her appearance on *The Tommy Tiernan Show*, in which O'Connor's honest account of living with Parkinson's was met with a groundswell of support from the Irish public.

"As part of Parkinson's Awareness Week in April, O'Connor launched a five-part podcast focusing on personal stories from the Irish Parkinson's community, inspiring others to talk about their illness, debunking the stigma and the myths around the disease and becoming an agent of change for how it, and those who live with it, are perceived."

I get out of my seat to a standing ovation as I'm called towards the stage. Hugging the editor, I reveal my schoolgirl error. "I just thought I was shortlisted."

"We wanted to keep it a surprise," she says. "So few things are." I walk up to the podium with my award and silently thank Mom before adjusting the microphone and acknowledging the support of *Irish Tatler*, the judges and everyone there that evening.

"I am humbled to be on this stage, in particular, after hearing the stories of all these incredible women," I say. When I was diagnosed with early-onset Parkinson's disease at age 47, a few months into my treatment, I knew I had a choice to make. I could play small and hide my condition or share my medical coming-out story and forge positive visibility for people with Parkinson's, especially young women like me.

"As I've said before, I never saw myself as an advocate, but I never saw myself dealing with an incurable brain disorder that affects my movement, mood and means of making a living. Parkinson's does not define me," I add, "but it is part of my narrative. And now my story belongs to others, because each time we share our personal stories, they become part of a collective anthology that facilitates change and serves a more insightful and equitable society."

I receive another standing ovation. Thankfully, this comes after my speech, as I'm at a loss for words. I feel like an accidental activist, a hero of circumstances. Ironically, the real catalyst in my story is Parkinson's. Why? Because it gives me no choice. If I want to see change, I have to change first. I have to let go of the life I once lived and the person I thought I was. I have to grieve now-defunct plans and rethink my goals. I have to accept the present to create space for my new self to emerge. I can sit back and do nothing or I can fight for my life – my short but beautiful life. I don't know what the future holds for my health. Only time will tell. Soon, days will fade with a distinct coolness as the pink sky prepares for dusk. Until then, we raise our glasses to mark the moment: this precious, fleeting moment.

It's after midnight and I'm ready to go home. Neil is, too.

"So, did you have the night of your life?" I ask him before we take our separate cabs. "No, not at all." He shakes his head. My heart sinks. "I believe that honour belongs to you. Well done again." I could scold him for his cheeky fake-out. Instead, I follow Mom's advice and let the good things come – no questions asked.

* * *

Lights off. Lamp on. Cup of tea beside me. I am tucked in bed replying to DMs and comments on Instagram when I hear the key in the door and "disarmed" announced by the alarm AI. Feet potter about in the kitchen; the fridge door opens, a cough, then the kettle. It's only been three years since I lived with Margaret, but it's comforting to know some things don't change when so much does. The pottering feet take measured steps upstairs towards my door. *Knock, knock.* "Are you awake?" asks the door, now slightly ajar.

"Come on in!" I scootch upright in the bed, back against the headboard.

"Hello, sibling, or should I say Catalyst of the Year?" Arms outstretched like kids playing aeroplanes, we reach for one another and land in a sisterly squeeze.

"I got your WhatsApp and saw the videos on Instagram. You must be so delighted." I hug my knees in tighter to make room for her to sit.

"It was a big shock. In typical form, I assumed I was a category nominee – not a winner. I probably could have cleared up any confusion with an email, but why make life easy? Speaking of which, I didn't think you'd be working on Saturday."

"Neither did I," she sighs. "I assumed I'd be home to congratulate you when you got back tonight, but I was delayed by over an hour. Someone took their life on a bridge overlooking the M50." My eyes widen.

"That was this afternoon," I chime in, "It was on the news!"

"There was still a big police presence and a motorway diversion in place. It's so sad. I found it all very unsettling."

"Puts things into perspective, doesn't it?" Our silent pause confirms it does.

"Do you have any plans for tomorrow?"

"I wanted to see Andy, but he texted me while I was on the train this morning to say he's too weak for visitors, so . . ."

"It must be so hard, Ams, I know. Think of how much energy it took for him to speak at your last visit."

She looks over at the cut-glass trophy. "I bet he's so proud of you, as we all are."

"I'll see him again before Christmas, no doubt. He'll cancel me if I don't bring him his annual box of rocky road." Margaret tries to force a smile, but her poker face is worse than mine.

She pats my upright shins. "Get some sleep. We can chat in the morning."

"Mags, I'm not in any rush tomorrow. Let's grab some breakfast if you're free."

* * *

November 19, 2023

Your space and place to thrive.

"For your next masterpiece," Catriona says, handing me a foolscap pad from the University of Galway, our alma mater.

I run my fingers over the words, which are positioned above a sketch of an ivy-clad quadrangle. "Even though it's our pearl anniversary, I'll take paper any day," I exclaim, genuinely excited with my gift.

Our friend group from college is celebrating 30 years together with a brunch at Sophie's rooftop restaurant, which boasts a 360-degree view of Dublin. This is my second time in the past week in the big smoke. A third violation and I might well lose my Cork passport.

It's not yet Christmas, but it certainly feels like it as Catriona plays Santa with the rest of the group. Seven of us out of ten, including Julie, are present and accounted for, bar Katherine, who is driving in thanks to a no-show Luas. Whatever about dating apps, public transport ghosting is the most egregious kind. It feels personal.

"I have to say, I'm impressed with the circular table," remarks Jen. "It's so much easier to chat with everyone than those big banquet things."

"Except if you're sitting on the inside, like Ams, and you have to pee." Iseult laughs with her entire body. We shared a house during our final year in college, so she is familiar with my petite bladder.

"I think it's time I change seats." I switch with Joanne for the side nearest the bathroom, congratulating myself on not spilling my coffee – a personal best, Parkinson's or not.

"Tell us all about your award, you sparkling diamond," Iseult demands with contagious glee. "We are so proud of you!"

What starts as a recap of the night develops into a deeper conversation about my Parkinson's experience. "Aside from the obvious physical tells, there are non-motor symptoms, like sleep disorders, pain and anxiety, while others are medication-related," I explain. "It can be quite lonely if you let it. That's why your community – whatever that looks like to you – is so important." It is too fresh to mention my weight (although it's hard not to notice), so I gloss over the subject, despite having stepped on the scales yesterday to discover I'm a few pounds lighter. "I'll be the first to admit, I'm not great at reaching out. I tend to rely on myself to my detriment, but it's a habit which I am unlearning."

Áine, flute of bubbles in hand, clears the heaviness. "That's the beauty of friendship: people come in and out of our lives at different times, and some return to roost. It's lovely to see it." And to that, we all cheers.

I look around the table at us women. We are all so different: married with children, divorced or single, well-off or just getting by, teachers, number crunchers, leaders and assistants. Regardless of how we move through the world, we are united by a kinship of three decades. If I take away anything from living with this disease, it's this: we are all stronger together, especially when times are tough.

Life is nothing but democratic, however unfair it might appear. All of us will get the twitch – that moment when the course of our lives unalterably changes. If we can look back on the ensuing series of events and see the same friends before *and* after, we are thriving.

And we are. Eggs Benedict, pancakes and a full Irish or three fill us up, along with overdue face-to-face chats and hours of too-loud laughter. Soon, we'll all have to go our separate ways. Julie is staying overnight for a work meeting in Ballsbridge tomorrow. I duly inform her that traitors are now subject to a toll upon using the Jack Lynch Tunnel.

I wait in Heuston station for the 5 p.m. train to Cork. For once, I have no luggage in tow except for my new notepad. I feel energised and hopeful. Possibilities seem possible. It doesn't feel like the other shoe is about to drop. Time passes in no time, and before I know it, I'm homeward bound. Once the whistle blows, I retrieve a pen from my bag and open the notepad, watching paper turn into pearls as I outline a new book – the story of my life: my life with Parkinson's.

CHAPTER TEN

Acceptance

Life goes on

December 2023–January 2024

I'M TAKING THE CHRISTMAS tree down early. That's not like me. Perhaps it's a dopamine dip or a case of the winter blues, but something is missing. There's no sparkle. There are no precious rescue breaths. It stands like a reminder of a feeling I can't access. Maybe this is how life goes. The older I get, the more I feel resigned to this prospect. Still, it's hard to put something away, to wrap delicate baubles of hope in tissue paper, taking care not to shatter them. It's hard to move on.

Andy dies early the next morning. I ring in the new year preparing to say goodbye to my friend: packing, distracting myself, desperate to fill time. On the day of his cremation, the sky is blue and the sun is high. A bewildered Mother Nature thinks it's spring, sending her daffodils and snowdrops to bloom, only to be snatched by the first frost. When the ceremony ends, the floor opens, allowing ashes to ashes and dust to dust as the earth takes him back home. Just like that. Gone. It's hard to believe I'll never see him again – in this lifetime, at least.

I think back on the gift my mom gave me as a teenager – remembering. And so, I speak Andy into the present with words, talking to him as if he's still here. I believe he is. Often, I sit on the leather foot stool facing the Eames chair and think out loud, unravelling a cat's cradle of menial problems. Always there for the small stuff as well as the big. That's him.

Days later, I receive an email confirming a publishing offer for my memoir about living with Parkinson's. Naturally, I accept. This is my chance to put the past few years into perspective, to share my vulnerabilities, cast off my fears and, in turn, give others permission to do the same.

Betrayed by excitement and joy, I am tempted to share the good news in the group chat, but Andy's passing is too recent, although he would be the first to berate me for biting my tongue. With my symptoms well-managed, I'm feeling the best I've felt since before my diagnosis. I have a present and a future tense. I'm the lucky one. I don't fight Parkinson's like I used to. Perhaps because I understand it better. I understand myself better, too. That's not to say I'm giving up. No, that's not me. I'm giving up the struggle, surrendering to what is and living life as best I can. That's all. What I *am* having trouble reconciling is how life goes on: this non sequitur of mourning and celebration – so beautifully cruel. I may not understand it, but I choose to accept it. And so, every day, I make an effort to mark the day. I chat with my family. I meet up with friends. I set the table. I remember Andy.

* * *

I sit cross-legged on my comfy chair, sequestered in the quiet of my apartment. Phone off, computer off – unplugged. Outside, 'new year, new you' messages search for willing ears.

Not mine. With my eyes closed, I remain still, listening to the hum of nothing. It feels nourishing, like a wholesome meal after a spell of fasting. I need it. My heart and mind are tired from the past year's push-pull and this year that is only starting.

I remember the smudge stick I left in the kitchen, a Christmas gift from Maureen, foraged from fallen Connemara heather and wild seasonal flowers. Placed in a shallow bowl next to the sink, I light the intertwined flotsam, blowing out the flame to create a billow of smoke, part of the ancient clearing ritual. Smudging the corners of the room, with front and back doors open, I set my intention to release the past and usher in the new, allowing nature to take back what I no longer need: the lessons learned, the losses mourned. I retreat to the comfy chair and wait as the smoke clears and peace fills the space before starting again. New year, different me. And that's OK. I won't make any resolutions: no stylish self-improvement plans. I just want to slow down. I want to stop fearing what's not in my power. I want to accept the future, whatever that looks like. I want release. That is my wish.

* * *

"My name is Annmarie. I'm here because I can't scream. Ironic, eh? And, yeah, I'm really fucking angry about that. The closest I get to screaming is crying. Don't get me wrong. A good cry occasionally is healthy, but Jesus, I don't know when to stop. Also, I'm blatantly gaslighting myself. My friend Andy passed away a few weeks ago from motor neurone disease. Ever watch someone you love die? It's like a sick reality show. Oh, and I have Parkinson's! I call it the middle child of emotional baggage. I'm too busy dealing with the symptoms and side effects to really let myself grieve. That would mean digging deep: wild, aggressive, banshee-style purging. Couldn't have that now, could we? What would the neighbours think? That's why I'm here, freezing my arse off on a Sunday morning. Out with the old and in with a dry robe, am I right? Almost 40 years living in Ireland and you'd think I'd learn to dress for the weather."

This is what my introduction sounds like in my head. When it comes time for me to share why I'm sitting around a fire on Garrylucas beach with 15 other women, my voice immediately breaks and I apologise for being emotional. Deep down, I know why I'm at a Scream Club. I need to find my voice. Not the one who writes and speaks for a living or the one who advocates for people with Parkinson's; I'm looking for the one who is muted by life's lawlessness. That one. Where is she? Stand up and be counted, for God's sake.

Instead, I sit and listen as bobble-hatted strangers show their soft underbellies, angry about social injustice, losing parents and partners – angry about life. I don't remember anyone's names, but I know them by their stories. For this short period of time, we are intimately connected, bound by trust.

I'm not even sure what voice activation is, but I commit to the morning meditation, listen to the drumming and keep my mind open. There are no words, just sound – empty syllables without meaning and, most importantly, without attachment. The metaphor isn't lost on me. Sometimes life just isn't fair. It helps to shout about it, to cry, but it also helps to move on. I seem to be having trouble with that despite my best efforts.

"Are you ready?" asks the club leader.

Ready as I'll ever be, I think to myself, following her warm maternal energy as she guides us to the water's edge.

I remember living as a kid on Long Island. I would spend my summers at Corey Beach, standing knee-deep in the waves as they broke over my body. The sheer force was invigorating. Once, a rip current caught me unawares, regurgitating me onto the shore with its salty jaws. For a split second, I blacked out. Weak, disoriented and unable to move, I wiped the sand from my mouth and slowly found my footing. People stared; some laughed. It didn't bother me. At that moment, I was fearless.

Now, not so much. Holding hands in a human chain, we prepare our lungs, tongues and vocal chords to unleash whatever is festering in our hearts and minds and just have done with it. Diaphragms engage, mouths open: something that passes for noise emerges from my throat's safety valve. *That'll be enough*, it tells me. Disappointed in myself, I join the others for cake and tea before the circle is closed, low-key envious of the genuine experiences of release around me. Some people vow to return, and those who attend the group regularly share insights. Everyone looks fresh and relieved. I want to be that person – the one who grieves recklessly. I tell myself once is enough. There's no need to go again, but I know this isn't true. Deprogramming my A-student will take time.

At home, I lie on the sofa, feeling relaxed and strangely at peace. With no distractions and no to-do list, I have a quiet 'a-ha!' moment. I think I'm using Andy's death as a proxy for my own grief: a survival mechanism so that I don't fall apart. Maybe the writing process will help sublimate some of these untapped feelings so that when it comes time to scream, I'll be fearless. Only time will tell. For now, I'll leave a key under the mat.

* * *

I have a year to write my memoir, which sounds like plenty of time, but in the context of managing work, health and a personal life, it's a precious commodity. A few days after I receive my publishing contract, Parkinson's Ireland asks me to chair their annual Education Conference. Keen to take part but also to honour my 2024 wishes, I decide to make it my singular charity focus for the year. Marking Parkinson's Awareness Week, the subject matter for this year's online forum is Parkinson's 40-plus symptoms, with special attention given to the role of emotional well-being in keeping healthy. For me, raising awareness is a way to give back to an organisation that continues to help me and those I know, but it's also a way for the Parkinson's community at large to shine a light on the complex side of the disease, which is often shrouded in stigma.

Whether a symptom of the disease or a side effect of medication, anxiety, depression and apathy is a common trifecta, not to mention the indignity and embarrassment often linked to experiencing an impulse control disorder or psychosis-like delusions or hallucinations. Only when we open dialogue on such matters, be it with friends and family or at events such as these, can we dismantle the power these emotions have over us. There, I'll get off my soapbox – for now. Not that I have any business standing on it in the first place.

At times, I feel like a fraud when it comes to discussing my interior world. I can chat about Parkinson's without feeling sad, broken or humiliated. The food noise in my head, though – that's a whole different TED Talk. Parkinson's happened to me. Food, however, is more nuanced.

There's shame in eating too much or too little. With personal agency comes self-blame, which often perpetuates the yo-yo cycle of overeating and restricting, not to mention the psychological fallout of gaining weight again: how quickly it goes back on, the fear of stepping on scales, trying to button a too-small pair of trousers that shouldn't fit me in the first place. This occupies as much head space as remembering to replenish my meds and keep on schedule with my daily Parkinson's routine.

Quite frankly, it's exhausting. To misquote a law of metaphysics, two objects cannot occupy the same space simultaneously. When it comes to my mental real estate, something's got to give. Since Parkinson's calls dibs on fixed tenancy rights, the food squatters from yesteryear face eviction. This will take time, but my patience is well-documented. The irony at the intersection of these two experiences is that without Parkinson's, my unhealthy eating habits would remain dormant without ever healing. Not that I give Parkinson's any credit; it doesn't deserve it, but fair is fair. In fact, I still feel self-indulgent talking about my body image, like it's a first-world problem or a side effect of privilege. These are extraneous voices that I internalise until now.

* * *

After her experience of being thwarted by the Luas at last November's college brunch, my friend Katherine decides to drive to meet me for a bite to eat this January afternoon. Making good on my promise to reach out more for help, I'm hoping she'll have some advice about my recent weight loss. As a librarian with an owl tattoo and oodles of wisdom, she invariably finds the perfect words to clarify a situation, so I'm all ears.

"Think of it as an artefact from the past," she says, holding up a salt cellar like an ancient relic, "something you discovered on a Parkinson's dig. This isn't who you are. It is a pattern that illuminates who you were at a point in time. Useful," she is keen to add, "insofar as it informs the present."

I nod in appreciation. "I never thought of it that way. It makes sense. There's a definite through line between the new medication reducing my appetite and certain . . . patterns resurfacing." The word "eating" gets stuck in my mouth.

"It's so insidious. At first, I didn't recognise it for what it was, until I did . . ."

My voice cracks. "I mean, I even went to my doctor to check what was happening, not realising I was partly the problem – trying to keep my Parkinson's under control, being the A-student, doing everything to the letter."

"And you were quick to do something about it," she points out. Katherine puts down her cutlery and leans in, fingers interlocked. "Look at you, talking about your health objectively and with curiosity. That's not to say it doesn't hurt, but the experience doesn't have the same hold over you it once had."

My eyes offer a silent "thank you" as I take a small bite of my lunch and digest her sensible counsel. "Sometimes I think Parkinson's is drawing attention to an unhealed part of my heart," I admit. "Like a frenemy who tells you the love of your life is getting married because she thinks 'you deserve to know'. It's like, 'Great, now what?' Do you thank the person or throw a drink in their face? I think the latter."

"Why waste a good glass of wine?" Katherine chuckles. "Remember, you are now a woman with more life lived than your college self. You are discerning, you know your trigger points and now you have the tools to apply that emotional salve should you need it. I believe in you. And you know you always have us to lean on."

Later that week, I call my dietitian about an unrelated matter, and she kindly mentions her friend, an intuitive eating counsellor who is setting up a practice in Cork, should I be interested in attending a session. I'm grateful. Although, it could be a few months before I look into this. Recognising not-so-healthy eating patterns is one thing; doing something about it is another.

I recall what Julie said last August when we sat at the kitchen table. "Life is messy, Annie." Those words resonate differently for me now. Like grief, life isn't linear; paths cross and worlds collide. We live in the aftermath of choices and experiences as we move towards the future. No one is immune. We know each other by our scars. For some, the marks will be permanent. For those more fortunate, it's a chance to reframe what life looks like. Maybe it's time I do something about the mess – to navigate the middle path between too much and too little. To do that, I must let go of the old version of myself and appreciate who I am today.

The irony? Having more with less is the premise of my two books, *The Happy Closet* and *The Happy Medium*. Whether that's a wardrobe of clothes you actually wear or cultivating personal satisfaction, both choices rely on learning how to have enough or be enough: radical self-acceptance, if you will.

"We are all goddesses!" you'll hear me cheer when anyone puts their body down. Meanwhile, I fail to spot my own red flags as my appetite shrinks and bones protrude through my clothes. Could it be that I am trying to control my Parkinson's, which is controlling me? Yes, it could, which is why I'm letting that part of me die. This is my life, after all. Radical self-acceptance: I'm finally learning what that means.

From the outside, my life looks relatively unchanged. I work in the same industry, have the same friends and live in the same place, but I'm not the same person, nor will I ever be. My skin is thicker, my intuition is sharper and my mind is wiser. I'm even sleeping through the night again. I still have trouble with fatigue and persistent gut issues. Not to mention the dyskinesia in my left shoulder and tremor in my right hand, which casually conspire against me when under stress. On occasion, the vibrations and body-popping make it look like

I'm auditioning for a breakdance crew – the girl who doesn't dance. Overall, this is a vast improvement compared to who I was at the time of my diagnosis, and that's good enough for me. My biggest win is being able to type again. As I write about my experience with Parkinson's, I realise how lucky I am to have a steady hand and to be able to share these intimate details with you.

Writing is healing. It's my palliative tool. I'm not one for regular journalling, but when I turn on my laptop and place my hands on the keyboard, a certain alchemy happens. Thoughts flow through my fingertips. At times, the words don't feel like mine. It's as if my conscious mind detaches momentarily, allowing my higher self to dig deep for flashes of insight, transmuting the base metals of my journey into gold.

I remember hearing on a podcast some time ago that once art is put out into the world, it no longer belongs to the writer, the painter or the actor. It now belongs to the audience. It is theirs to fête, to critique or to flat-out ignore. The artist's job is to let go and allow. Starting over isn't easy, but neither is harking back to the past – unless, as my friend Katherine says, it is an artefact that helps you grow. Soon, this book will belong to you, but the healing will belong to *us* – a connection over geography and time. Such is the beauty of art, and for that, I thank you.

March 2024

"I'm stuffed. Next time, we should probably share one," I suggest, "and order a few sides instead." Julie sighs in agreement. The Neapolitan pizza at Palmento is legendary. So is the time I put chilli oil on Julie's goat cheese calzone. Why people allow me to season their food is anyone's guess. The trust is appreciated but also wildly misplaced.

Without warning, there is an all too familiar noise. The roof sounds like it is being pebble-dashed or accosted by light gunfire. "Hailstones," we conclude in tandem, shaking our heads as if disappointment will dissipate the lousy weather.

"Seville can't come soon enough," I moan. "Only one month until sunshine." Our server asks us if we'd like to look at the dessert menu. It would be rude not to try the tiramisu for two. We're not those kinds of people.

"I meant to ask, Annie. When you and Neil travel together, do people ever think you're a couple?"

"Always. It's weird because he's like my brother. We went to Cambodia a lifetime ago and everyone called us Mr and Mrs Neil. In fact, we had dinner one night in this little restaurant where they set up a separate beachside table with fairy lights and music unbeknownst to us. The tide was coming in and our table sank into the sand. The hem of my dress was soaking up so much water, I had to keep ringing it out."

"What did you do?"

"What *could* we do? They thought we were Mr and Mrs Neil – the world's most platonic couple."

"Do you ever think that's why you haven't met anyone special yet, you both being so close?"

"I don't necessarily think so," I muse. "I do think that there's an intimacy with friendships that you don't always find in romantic connections. Neil knows everything about me and my Parkinson's – *as do you*. Maybe I should be more aware of it when I start dating again."

"Are you thinking of it?" Her voice twinkles with expectation. I shrug and offer a non-committal "maybe". Julie knows that 'bouncing back' is a term reserved for rubber bands, not humans with hearts and bodies that break easily. It could take time for me to come full circle.

"Now that my symptoms are levelling out, I feel more accepting of the status quo. This is me, like it or not. Chances are my nervous system *will* pitch a fit again – and again. I can't put my good enough on silent, afraid that someone will want something better." Our tiramisu arrives, which we make short work of before settling the bill and dodging the next hail shower.

Huddling under an umbrella, we walk together to the intersection at the top of the road, both of us ready to go our separate ways. "It's weird being in my fifties, Jules. I'm officially an older woman, but I still feel so young."

"That's a good sign, surely." She squeezes me goodbye. "It means your sparkle is back."

I spot the bus stop across the road where, not too long ago, I broke down on the phone to Margaret with a pillbox in my hand, convinced my life was over. It feels like a stranger's memory. A sigh of relief follows.

"I'm turning a corner, I think, Jules."

"No, Annie," she says, crossing the road. "You're going straight ahead."

April 2024

It's time to go away, to vacate our everyday lives, if only for a few days. That's what we do, Neil and I. Andy's absence makes me more intentional about spending time with friends and keen to put the 'extra' in life's 'ordinary'.

We decide on Seville, with its Andalusian architecture, tapas and guaranteed sunshine. Nothing in life is a sure thing, not least the weather, but a late-April visit should tip the odds in our favour. After another winter where we baby-name storms and colour-code weather warnings, we could use the heat.

Despite this truism, I spend the days leading up to our mini break stalking weather sites and I discover a cold front is due over the south of Spain on the exact five days of our trip. I remind myself that 20 degrees with passing showers is considered an Irish summer. Neither Balearic nor Baltic, it is, in fact, just right.

On arrival, we make a pact to ignore the YouTube videos touting the same tourist-filled 'hidden gems', choosing instead to explore the city's food markets and second-hand haunts, taking shortcuts through brightly painted side streets and sitting on our balcony as the evening sun briefly illuminates the Gothic cathedral, leaving an ombré flourish in its wake.

Neil, who is travelling from Dublin, arrives the night before and is there to greet me when my cab arrives early the next morning. I leave to get snacks for our Airbnb before we head to MaríaTrifulca, on the Triana side of the Guadalquivir River bridge, for dinner. With 10 per cent battery on my Android and a vague idea of how to get to the Mercado de Triana, I allow overconfidence to lead the way as I wander its cobbled streets in the opposite direction. Truth be told, I have Google Maps open and still can't find it, which elicits mild anxiety, enough to realise I am completely off course, with pidgin Spanish and a bout of Parkinson's fatigue kicking in. I don't look lost, I look drunk – unable to string a sentence together and quite willing to take a nap on the nearest flat surface. I recognise a tourist bodega with flamenco paraphernalia outside and I realise I'm only 500 metres away from home and a pre-dinner power nap.

By the end of the trip, I'm better accustomed to my surroundings and can find my way around the city alone without relying on Neil to be my satnav. That's when I notice something peculiar – a dearth of oranges. I spot splattered remains on the sidewalk from the trees lining Calle San Fernando alongside the university. Aside from that, the trees are conspicuously bare, bar a few stalwarts.

We're too late, I think, gutted we hadn't thought to book our flights earlier. The season for Seville oranges finishes mid-February, with those poised for marmalade status picked in November and December. The unchosen are left to spoil on the branches. Although not fit for bittersweet jelly, their beauty never fades; even when they detach from the branch and fall to the ground, their pectin releases an acrid smell, serving as a reminder of life coming around again. The street sweepers gather up most of the decaying skins for compost. It's advisable not to pick any defectors you see on the street as, technically, even the skins belong to the city council.

The season might be over, but I am determined to see an orange tree in full bloom before leaving Seville. I take a walk through the Jewish Barrio in Santa Cruz. Amid its whitewashed alleyways and quirky artisan shops, I spot an unassuming building with a sign above its cast iron doors: *Hospital des Venerables Sacerdotes*. Seville's Venerable Hospital, I discover, is a 17th-century institution once used as a care home for ageing and poor priests after the 1647 plague in Seville. I pay €12 for entry and a self-guided tour device I don't use. My attention travels elsewhere. Planted in a semi-circle within the courtyard's central patio are six orange trees with fruit-laden branches. *Were they planted for medicinal properties or their aromatic blossoms?* I wonder. The Chinese and Arabs considered them a symbol of happiness. To think that a tree, originally from the Himalayas, can still grow, even when propagated on foreign soil. I'm in awe at such resilience.

Despite being flanked by the palace of the Royal Alcázar and equally majestic Plaza de España, a welfare building harbouring overripe oranges is, without doubt, the highlight of my trip. Riches so simple fill me with excitement, which makes looking at life a lot easier, given its challenges. This is one of those riches: a moment of joy and awe that overrides my chaotic nervous system and allows me to forget, albeit briefly, that I have Parkinson's.

I return to our Airbnb with a sense of satisfaction. Neil and I pack the rest of our things before heading out for our last meal of baby clams and braised pork cheek at a neighbourhood restaurant. Soon, it'll be time to go. Time to return to the everyday, the expected – those beautiful banalities that keep me balanced. For how long, I don't know. Then again, who does? Life doesn't provide timelines, and I don't do guessing games.

All I know is that when the twitch comes again, *and it will*, I won't be ready. No one ever is. Like a silent cataclysm, it will leave me to struggle under the burden of 'why?' It will break me down and force me to make changes so that I may build myself up. That's its job; it's nothing personal. What we must remember is that we always have a choice. We can remain bitter, bruised and out of season, or we can gather what has fallen, that once-fragrant flesh, and start over – the same life, just different.

Epilogue

July 2024

PATRICIA HOLDS THE THREE-TIER cake for dear life on the *Adventurer*, while Maureen and I are poised as marker players should we hit a wave. It's Margaret's 60th birthday and we're heading to Inishbofin to celebrate, hence the hydrangea-shaped confection.

Grateful for the flat crossing, we order cappuccinos and flat whites at the Saltbox when we hit dry land, gabble about weekend plans and let Mom know we're on our way.

"Here, allow me." An outstretched arm spots mine, long but shaky, attempting a group selfie. "It's lovely to see you sisters together again," says the food truck owner as I hand her my phone.

We find our family portrait poses as the sun dismisses idle threats from passing clouds. *Snap.* I thank her for the kind gesture – a moment of certainty captured in a world of questions.

I look at the photo on my phone: the five of us, arms around each other, balancing takeaway coffees, with squints and smiles. As moments go, this deserves a frame. Together again, for the time being, anyway. That's all that matters. Twitch. Blink and you'll miss it.

Acknowledgements

I WROTE *TWITCH* AT my kitchen table – where I work, eat with friends and family, open my post, unpack my groceries and pay my bills. A rectangular piece of granite supported by wooden legs and iron braces; it is my apartment's most important piece of furniture. The overhead lighting isn't great. The too-deep chairs need pillow props and I always seem to hit my knee on one of the beams when crossing my legs. This is life, or at least where life happens – my life.

When editing the manuscript, I noticed how often the kitchen table (mine and that of my youth) appears in my story, especially at pivotal moments. I began to think of it as my strong yet silent character, someone I could trust with my hopes and fears, until I looked closer at the scenes. Those people already exist. Some feature in the book and others don't, but they are all central to my life. My kitchen table, as it so happens, is more so an unintentional device for connection and kinship, a place where these relationships are nurtured, celebrated and strengthened. With that, I'd like to thank the following people who made this book a reality. May you always have a seat at my table.

My mother Irene, and my four sisters, Margaret, Catherine, Maureen and Patricia for their love and support.

My two Auntie Margarets for their kind help.

My editor Vickie, and the *Irish Examiner* for their empathy and encouragement.

Everyone at Parkinson's Ireland, especially Lisa, Richelle, Jerome and Marie.

My GP and the neurology department at Cork University Hospital.

Dr Sweeney for being such an instrumental guiding force.

Julie for a lifetime of friendship.

My readers and confidants, Katherine, Julie (Jules), Neil and Vickie, your feedback is deeply appreciated.

Deirdre, my publisher and the team at Eriu and Bonnier Books.

Miki for the cover photo.

My dear friend Neil, you're a rare find. I say *everyone should have a Neil*, but not everyone does. I'm lucky to have you in my life.

A special and heartfelt thank you to Andy's family.

For the purposes of this book, I relied on my diary entries, text messages, emails, calendars, my memories and those of my friends and family.

Annmarie x

About Annmarie

Annmarie O'Connor is a fashion editor, bestselling author, TEDx speaker and well-known media contributor. In 2021, she was diagnosed with early-onset Parkinson's disease, an incurable neurodegenerative condition, broadly affecting movement and mental health. She now uses her platform to spread awareness and bring about positive social change. Originally from New York, she now lives in Cork, Ireland.